A History
of the Catechumenate
The First Six Centuries

by Rev. Michel Dujarier

Translated from the French
by Edward J. Haasl

D1556964

Sadlier
A Division of William H. Sadlier, Inc.
New York
Chicago
Los Angeles

Translator's Note

The scriptural citations are taken from *The Holy Bible: Revised Standard Version*, 1952, Collins, Fontana Books.

When suitable and authoritative translations of the patristic texts could be found, they were used and are so cited in the notes. Otherwise, the translations are from the French texts cited by the author.

Home Office:
11 Park Place
New York, N.Y. 10007
ISBN: 0-8215-9327-7
123456789/9

Contents

Introduction	5
Abbreviations	8
The Major Options of the	
New Testament Era	9
Some Norms from the Initial Period	11
A Perennial Objection	14
The Requirements for Admission to	
Baptism	19
The Jewish Practices	22
Notes	27
The Structuring of the	
Catechumenate (Second-Third Centuries)	29
An Abiding Concern for	
Pastoral Authenticity	31
In Rome ca. 150	35
In Egypt ca. 190-200	41
In North Africa ca. 200-210	44
In Rome ca. 215	48
In Egypt and Palestine ca. 230-240	55
In Syria and Palestine ca. 250	64
At the Dawn of the Fourth Century	69
Notes	72
The Vicissitudes of the	
Catechumenate (Fourth-Sixth Centuries)	77
The New Problems	79
The Permanent Concern for Authenticity	85
The Catechumenate from 350 to 420	91

4

Evaluation of the Fourth and Fifth
Centuries   107
Conclusion   112
Notes   115

*Appendix I: Can a History of the
Catechumenate Be Written?*   121
General Survey   122
Special Studies   124
Notes   128

*Appendix II: Decline and Revival
of the Catechumenate: Sixth to the
Twentieth Century*   131
The Eclipse of the Catechumenate   133
Modern Missionary Efforts   136
The Conciliar Renewal   140
Notes   143

Introduction
By Christiane Brusselmans

THIS book is not a formal research study concocted in a calm and disinterested ivory tower. Michel Dujarier is not a dispassionate observer of his subject; he searches for the practical truth of the matter in order to apply it to his immediate concerns: conversion, faith, and baptism as the seal and sign of that conversion and faith. And these concerns are not abstractions: they are focused on and have derived from the very real catechumens Fr. Dujarier is working with in his catechumenal communities in West Africa.

There is a long tradition in the Church for this kind of pastoral writing, a tradition that includes the Evangelists and the Fathers of the Church. It is a pragmatic tradition in the best sense of the word: speculation, research, argument, polemic—all are directed to the very practical and immediate ends of preaching the Word of God, of making it comprehensible, and of allowing it to work its converting force.

And when the early Church preached, it did not presume to think that the bare announcement of the message of salvation was sufficient. It followed up the initial reception of the kerygma with a structured, supervised, and extended formation period and initiation into the fullness of the mysteries of Christ. The catechumenate was one of the first institutions the Church structured. It makes a difference what a Christian believes and how that belief is lived. And such living is an art that must be learned: we have to learn to believe, to love, to see, to change our ways in life. One is not born a Christian, one becomes a Christian.

The early Church saw the convert's first burst of enthusiasm for what it was: a fragile reality that was apt to evaporate as quickly as it appeared. The new converts had to be taught, tested, and brought to maturity. The ultimate test for sincerity and authenticity was always moral conversion.

But once the Church became socially and legally accepted, other reasons arose for joining it. Among them were social acceptance, professional advancement, political preferment, and, all too often, simply socio-cultural habit. At the dawn of the fourth century, with the Edict of Milan (313), Christendom, a political and geographical entity, was born and, along with it, baptism was often cheapened. Instead of being a sign of sin rejected, of faith accepted, of conversion accomplished, it was all too often experienced as granting citizenship in the empire

But neither the idea nor the practice of extended periods of formation were lost to the Church. The catechumenate was transferred to the monasteries, convents, and seminaries. And the ministries were also transferred to the "experts" who had profited from the formation period. The laity tended to become mere passive recipients of sacraments or observers of a process in which they were not personally involved. No longer were they called to exercise their ministries in the Church. These were performed for them.

The rediscovery of the dignity of the laity and the elaboration of an authentic theology of ministry prepared the way for renewal. The crucial task of nurturing and expanding the Body of Christ can only be done effectively if a variety of complementary ministries are reestablished and exercised in the Church. All this was given eloquent expression by the Second Vatican Council.

Father Dujarier sees the clear analogy between the situation of the Church today—isolated and often ignored in a secular society—and that of the ancient Church in the Roman world of the early centuries (1-3). Like the ancient Church, the Church today cannot count on society and its institutions to help convey the message of Christ—if, indeed, it ever could.

The Church must take care of its own and see to its future generations. For this, the re-establishment of the adult catechumenate is perhaps one of the most important pastoral developments of the post-Vatican II era. Father Dujarier's experience with the catechumenate has been both practical and creative. What he gives us here are the roots and historical background for that experience.

I know of no better study of the history of the catechumenate in the early Church existing today.

Bishops, pastors, priests, deacons, and religious as well as liturgists and catechists will find it extremely helpful. This book could also serve as a text in university courses and in professional schools of theology, liturgy, and religious education.

Finally, researchers will find in this book, and especially in Appendix I, valuable indications and bibliographical references to carry on further study and research in this area.

Christiane Brusselmans
Pentecost 1979

8
Abbreviations

AAS   Acta Apostolicae Sedis, Rome.

ACW   Ancient Christian Writers, Westminster, Maryland, The Newman Bookshop.

CCL   Corpus Christianorum, series latina.

ES   Collection Les Ecrits des Saints, Ed. du Soleil Levant, Namur.

FC   Fathers of the Church, Washington, D.C., The Catholic University of America Press.

GCS   Die Griechische Christlichen Schriftsteller, Leipzig, Berlin.

LC   Collections Lettres Chrétiennes, collection, Ictus, Paris.

PG   Patrologie Grecque, Migne, Paris.

PL   Patrologie Latine, Migne, Paris.

PLS   Patrologie Latine, suppléments.

PO   Patrologie Orientale.

SC   Sources Chrétiennes, Ed. du Cerf, Paris.

ST   Studi e Testi, collection, Vatican City.

TD   Textes et Documents pour l'Étude Historique du Christianisme, collection, H. Hemmer and P. Lejay, Paris.

The Major Options
of the New Testament Era

WITHOUT attempting to locate an institutional catechumenate in the New Testament—in fact there was none—it is still useful to see how the Church, from its very beginning, placed certain requirements on the reception of the sacraments and of baptism in particular.[1] Even though the Acts of the Apostles is primarily concerned with the life of the Spirit, the manifestations of the Spirit in the first communities, and the charisms that led people to Jesus, it also contains solid references to pastoral practice, which was also moved by the Spirit.

Some Norms
from the Initial Period

AN attentive reading of the Acts and the epistles shows us that the Church has always acted with circumspection when it admitted someone to an ecclesial office or to a consecrated state. It demanded certain qualities of the candidate and even a time of probation so that the candidate's aptitude could be judged effectively.

These demands, which existed from the very beginning, would soon be given a rather detailed codification, as can be seen when one compares the Pauline Epistles to Acts. And before a decision was made to admit someone, those responsible often appealed to the witness of the community.

From the beginning of the Church, ministers were chosen with care.

The account of the election of the first deacons outlines the qualities required of the candidates and specifies the intervention of the Christian community. In fact, it was the brothers who chose them and who witnessed to their aptitude. Then they were presented to the responsible authorities who ordained them.

> And the twelve summoned the body of the disciples and said, ". . . pick out from among you seven men of good repute, full of the Spirit and of wisdom, whom we may appoint to this duty. . . ." And what they said pleased the whole multitude, and they chose Stephen, a man full of faith and of the Holy Spirit, and Philip, and Prochorus, and Ni-

> canor, and Timon, and Parmenas, and Nico-
> laus, a proselyte of Antioch. These they set
> before the apostles, and they prayed and laid
> their hands upon them (Acts 6:2-6).

The choice of preachers was equally meticulous. Even Paul, who began to preach after his conversion (Acts 9:20-22), had to be admitted by the authorities after having been presented by Barnabas, a member of the community who was able to guarantee his conversion, his baptism, and even the orthodoxy of his teaching (Acts 9:26-28). In the same way, Paul took Timothy with him only upon the recommendation of the brothers (Acts 16:2-3).

Thirty years later, there is the same degree of seriousness with regard to more precise requirements. The Church, which had organized itself, established specific regulations.[2]

A bishop had to satisfy a set of clearly defined requirements (I Tim 3:2-7). Deacons, too, were chosen on the basis of detailed criteria and were subject to a period of probation during which they showed that they did in fact possess the required virtues.

> Deacons likewise must be serious, not dou-
> ble-tongued, not addicted to much wine, not
> greedy for gain; they must hold the mystery
> of the faith with a clear conscience. And let
> them also be tested first; then if they prove
> themselves blameless let them serve as dea-
> cons (I Tim 3:8-10).

Widows at the time also constituted a group that was recognized by the Church. But only those women were admitted who could furnish the witness of good behavior in accordance with the established criteria (I Tim 5:9-11).

Are not the same basic requirements of probation and aptitude also present in the baptismal discipline?

Ever since the Spirit of Pentecost has erupted into the world, the new People of God has been living in an eschatological time. Everything is grace and it does seem that, in the time of the Holy Spirit, there is no longer a place for long novitiates. However real this affirmation may be, it ought not to cause us to forget that, even at the beginning, the Church did not confer baptism lightly.

A Perennial Objection

How often has the reading of the Acts of the Apostles raised a certain doubt in the minds of pastors about the necessity of catechumenal stages? If the Christians of the Pentecost and the Ethiopian eunuch were baptized so quickly, why should one want to be so exigent today?

The objection is not new. There have always been those who have tried to justify with Luke's report a too hasty admission to baptism. The Fathers refuted this position: far from presenting a difficulty, the Lucan texts reveal the fundamental elements we shall be dealing with.

First, Tertullian:

> If Philip so "easily" baptized the chamberlain, let us reflect that a manifest and conspicuous evidence that the Lord deemed him worthy had been interposed. The Spirit had enjoined Philip to proceed to that road: the eunuch himself, too, was not found idle, nor as one who was suddenly seized with an eager desire to be baptized; but, after going up to the temple for prayer's sake, being intently engaged on the divine Scripture, was thus suitably discovered.[3]

In the same sense, St. Augustine argues that this passage from Acts definitely does not signify that one can be baptized without preparation. Quite the contrary. Philip not only performed all the essential liturgical rites, he also took time to educate the eunuch. He omitted nothing of "what pertains to the habits and morals of the faithful as well as what pertains to faith."

> If, however, Scripture is silent and dismisses the rest of what Philip talked over with the eunuch as understood and taken for granted, the words "Philip baptized him" imply that everything was fulfilled which, for the sake of brevity, may be passed over in Scripture, but which, nevertheless, we know from the unbroken chain of tradition must have been carried out. Likewise, where it says that Philip had preached the Lord Jesus to the eunuch, there must be no doubt that the ensuing catechism embraced all the necessary instruction on the duties and proper mode of living for one who believes in the Lord Jesus. To preach Christ consists in declaring not only what must be believed about Him, but also what precepts must be observed by one hoping for membership in the unity of the Body of Christ.[4]

It is sufficient to reread the text of Acts to realize how all the guarantees were provided. Luke sketches clearly the dispositions of the postulant: he is already a believer since he came on pilgrimage and studied the Bible (Acts 8:27-28), and the quality of his dispositions was confirmed by the witness of God himself (8:26,29). The candidate had made a long personal journey (8:34) and, after having listened to a Christo-centric biblical catechesis (8:35), he could proclaim his faith, and thus open the way to baptism.

Nevertheless, the author of Acts still presents the event as something exceptional. His intention seems to have been to show the spontaneity and intensity of the conversion of the heart and particularly the power of the Spirit, who intervenes miraculously.[5]

St. Augustine gathered together the arguments of those who believed in baptism without preparation in the New Testament to show their inanity. Thus, with regard to the three thousand converts at Pentecost, he stresses that moral catechesis was not forgotten and that the biblical text itself is already a refutation of those who would baptize unworthy candidates:

> In the very words of Peter . . . they have the source from which they could have been admonished, if they had cared to study them diligently. When he had said: "Repent and be baptized every one of you in the name of Jesus Christ for the forgiveness of your sins; and you will receive the gift of the Holy Spirit " . . . the writer of the book immediately added the words: "And with very many other words he bore witness, and exhorted them, saying: Save yourselves from this perverse generation. Now they who received his word accepted it eagerly and believed and were baptized, and there were added that day about three thousand souls." Who does not here understand that, with the "very many other words" which were omitted by the writer for the sake of brevity, Peter with strong appeal had urged them to tear themselves away from this perverse generation, since this very thought is itself concisely contained in the many words with which he was urging it upon them?[6]

The fundamental requirements for admission to

baptism emerge from this first baptismal narrative (Acts 2:37-41). Contrary to the opinion that sees baptism here being administered without preparation, there is a procedure that is already rather developed, even if later editing could have projected back more evolved customs than those of the time when the events took place. In particular, there is the journey of serious conversion, which is actively manifested in stages.[7]

Furthermore, there is an error of interpretation that is often made with regard to Acts 2:41. When reading "and there were added that day about three thousand souls," one thinks spontaneously that "that day" refers to the day of Pentecost itself. Obviously, however, "that day" is an eschatological term. What is being said is that those who received his word were baptized; "that day" is the day of baptism and not the day of Pentecost. "That day" stresses the eschatological role of baptism, the day when God gathers to his people those of all languages and races.

It does not seem, therefore, that the Apostles were always quick to baptize, even if they did do so sometimes.[8] However this may be, the texts insist on the necessity of discernment. It can even be affirmed that, very soon, ecclesiastical discipline came to be structured more and more firmly on the basis of the fundamental requirements one can perceive from the very beginning of Acts on.

The Epistle to the Hebrews gives witness to this when it reminds the Christians of their formation period when they could only digest milk, when they received the "elementary doctrines of Christ," the "foundation." This period must have been taken quite seriously, for one could not return to it after baptism, when one must eat solid food:

For though by this time you ought to be teachers, you need someone to teach you again the first principles of God's word. You need milk, not solid food; for everyone who lives on milk is unskilled in the word of righteousness, for he is a child. But solid food is for the mature, for those who have their faculties trained by practice to distinguish good from evil.

Therefore let us leave the elementary doctrines of Christ and go on to maturity, not laying again a foundation of repentance from dead works and of faith toward God, with instruction about ablutions, the laying on of hands, the resurrection of the dead, and eternal judgment. And this we will do if God permits (Heb 5:12–6:3).

The Requirements for Admission to Baptism

FROM the Pentecost event on, faith is obviously the central element of conversion. This faith is progressively "Christian": it is not just belief in God as creator (like the pagans) or even just in the God of the Old Testament (like the Jews), but in the God of Jesus Christ. The oldest letter of the New Testament states this explicitly and points the way for converts:

> For they themselves report concerning us what a welcome we had among you, and how you turned to God from idols, to serve a living and true God, and to wait for his Son from heaven, whom he raised from the dead, Jesus who delivers us from the wrath to come (I Thess 1:9-10).

The narrative of the baptisms at Pentecost even indicates two moments in the access to faith, two periods marked by two thresholds.

First, there is the kerygmatic announcement (Acts 2:14-36). This period, in which the mystery of the risen Christ is proclaimed, terminates in the first threshold: "Now when they heard this they were cut to the heart, and said to Peter and the rest of the apostles, 'Brethren, what shall we do?' " (Acts 2:37). This almost ritual question occurs again and again in the kerygmatic context. It manifests the first conversion that allows the taking of a step toward baptism. Indeed, what is involved is a real and profound faith, a faith prepared to move on to action.[9]

But the faith was not yet stabilized. It had to be consolidated by more thorough teaching, by the "many other words" of which Augustine stresses the importance. Once across the first threshold, there was a certain period of catechesis (Acts 2:38-40). This time of instruction and formation ends with the second threshold, where it is a question of determining if the candidates have applied the message in their lives, if they have "received his word" (Acts 2:41), that is to say, if they have obeyed Christ in practice, if they have changed their behavior enough to be admitted to baptism.

Access to baptism thus already seems to involve two distinct stages and two thresholds. Even though these two thresholds were very close to each other at the beginning, the redactor of the narrative clearly delineates them: an initial evangelization issuing in an act of faith—global but real since one's very existence is involved—and a more detailed catechesis that must be translated into concrete acts.

The narrative of the baptism of Cornelius (Acts 10:1-11, 18) is even clearer. Its structure suggests what could have been the baptismal stages when the Acts were compiled in the last third of the first century.[10]

The various descriptions we have of the scene have an introductory section, which is situated outside of a house (10,17, and 25). This is, in effect, the first stage, that of the approach to someone in authority who asks the traditional question: "What is your motive?" (10:21,29). The candidate replies by indicating that he is "just and fears God" (10:22,30) and by asking to be admitted to catechesis (10:22,33). This request is supported by guarantees: the witness of the angel (10:4,31), the three envoys (10:22), and the Jewish community (10:22). And, as appears from other, later texts, admission to catechesis is signified by the entry into the house (10:23,27).

Then the catechesis proper takes place (10:34-43). It is centered on Christ (10:36), whose lordship is demonstrated by the events that extend from the baptism by John to the resurrection appearances (10:37-41). The guarantee is provided by the preachers (10:42). Such instruction is intended to awaken full faith in Christ and through it to lead to baptism (10:43).

If this faith is manifest, the baptism can take place. But its quality must first be verified. In Cornelius's particular case, when the "six brethren" did not dare to render a favorable opinion, it was necessary for God himself to provide the witness (15:8) by sending his Spirit (10:44; 11:15). Faced with this incontestable sign, the community decided to baptize (10:44-48).

The narratives of Acts give indications of a double examination bracketing the period of catechesis. These indications are reinforced by two things: this structure became the normal one a hundred years later, and it already existed in certain contemporary Jewish practices.

The Jewish Practices

THE religious currents that flourished during the New Testament epoch, especially Judaism and Essenism, can also contribute to our study to the degree that some of their customs could have influenced Christian institutions around the years 70-100, that is, when the Church was compelled to adopt more structured forms.

The Essenes

Some authors such as A. Benoit think that the Essenes exercised an influence on Christianity but less on its origins than on its subsequent evolution.[11] If a rather large number of Essenes did indeed convert to Christianity after the catastrophe of 70, they could well have contributed some of the principles of organization of their community to the Church. I shall point out here only some of the striking analogies between the stages of initiation in the Qumran community and those in the first Christian communities.

The recent discoveries at Qumran have confirmed and augmented what was known already from Josephus about their system of admission, which consisted of the following stages:

1. The postulant is first subjected to *one year of probation,* during which he practices the new lifestyle, but outside the community:

> A candidate anxious to join their sect is not immediately admitted. For one year, during

which he remains outside the fraternity, they prescribe for him their own rule of life, presenting him with a small hatchet, the loin-cloth already mentioned, and white raiment.

2. He then does a *novitiate of two years* during which he can participate progressively in certain rites, but not yet in all of them:

> Having given proof of his temperance during the probationary period, he is brought into closer touch with the rule and is allowed to share the purer kind of holy water, but is not yet received into the meetings of the community. For after this exhibition of endurance, his character is tested for two years more, and only then, if found worthy, is he enrolled in the society.[12]

This information suggests two important observations. First, we are dealing here with a progressive initiation that reminds one of the catechumenal stages that are reported by Hippolytus of Rome, as we shall soon see. In addition, each of these stages is considered as a time of formation and experimentation. To be admitted to them, one had to submit to "tests," particularly with regard to morals and life-style.

The Qumran documents complete the description given by Flavius Josephus.[13] They specify that the passage from the postulancy to the novitiate was subject to the approval of the entire community. Each of the two years of the novitiate ended with an examination of the candidate, the passage to the superior degree depending on the opinion of the members who were charged with judging his aptitude.

Absolute sincerity of conversion was considered to

be a *sine qua non*. As Tertullian and Origen would later state, the bathing with water is inefficacious when the individual refuses to live according to the law of God. And with regard to hypocrites, the rule of the Qumran community is severe: "Let such a man not enter the water to proceed to the purification of the men of Sanctity, for one is not purified if he is not converted from his evil, since he is impure among all the transgressors of His word."[14]

The Admission of Proselytes

Since some elements of our Christian baptismal rite could have been affected by Jewish customs, it is useful to consider how the converted pagans were admitted to the community of the Old Covenant.[15]

Baptism of proselytes, written codification of which dates from the first half of the second century, was already in force at the end of the first century. The rite mentions a very serious entrance examination during which three rabbis tried to ascertain why the pagan wanted to join the Chosen People. They tested the quality of the conversion and even tried to discourage the convert by reminding him of the persecution of the Jews throughout the world.

> If in these days a man arrives to become a proselyte, he must be addressed as follows: "For what reason do you want to become a proselyte? Do you not know that Israel in this time is persecuted, oppressed, humiliated, and crushed, and that the suffering overwhelms her?" If he answers: "I know and I am not worthy," he is accepted forthwith.[16]

If the candidate remains firm in his decision, he is

admitted to instruction. It is only when he knew God's commandments and the punishments associated with them as well as the prospect of the world to come that he could be circumcised and baptized in the presence of two or three witnesses.

> If he has accepted, he is circumcised immediately . . . As soon as he is healed, he is baptized. Then, two knowledgeable men must stay by his side and inform him of some minor and major commandments. When he emerges from the immersion, he is considered in all respects as an Israelite.[17]

In this first period, the Church, which remained faithful to Jewish customs and to the Jewish community (Acts 3-15), was steeped in these rites and customs. It is not surprising that traces of them should have been left.

Some authors hesitate to admit an influence of Jewish rites on Christian rites. Still, it seems to me that there must have been such an influence, at least in Judeo-Christian milieux, both in the West and in the East. One indication of this is the appellation "proselyte of Christ " that is applied to catechumens in some texts of the second and even the third century.[18]

Still more than entrance into the Old Covenant, entrance into the New Covenant is a gift of God to which one must respond in all sincerity.

This brief survey of the New Testament has shown that the primitive Church only admitted to the sacraments of initiation those in whom it observed the faith of conversion and whose manner of life it had tested throughout the period of catechesis. It did not admit anyone without preparation, without tests, without guarantees. Thus entry into Christianity was not done in a way that departed from the customs of the contemporary religious communities of Judaism even though, during the initial years, the prospect of an imminent Parousia led the first Christians to accelerate the stages.

In the New Testament, there are probably more indications of a progressive initiation than the study of the admission of proselytes and of the novitiate of the Essenes allows us to identify.

At the end of the first century, the catechumenate did not yet exist as a settled institution, but the catechumenal reality was lived. From Pentecost on, the same requirements remained in force and, to preserve the purity of the community, they were soon translated into more clearly defined pastoral practices. The fruit to be harvested can already be seen in the seeds that were being sown. Growth began and maturity would be attained in the first half of the third century.

Notes

[1]Cf. Michel Dujarier, *Le Parrainage des adultes aux trois premiers siècles de l'Eglise, Parole et mission* 4, Paris, 1962, pp. 68-171.

[2]Cf. J. Dauvillier, *Les temps apostoliques: 1er siècle*, Sirey, Paris, 1970.

[3]Tertullian, *De bapt.* 18, 20. *The Writings of Quintus Sept. Flor. Tertullianus*, vol. I, Translated by Alexander Roberts and James Donaldson, *Ante-Nicene Christian Library*, vol. XI, Edinburgh, Clark, 1869, p. 252.

[4]Augustine, *De fide et op.*, 9, 14; *St. Augustine, Treatises on Marriage and Other Subjects*, trans. by Charles T. Wilcox, FC 27, p. 237.

[5]In the narrative of the baptism of the eunuch, the intention is not to give an example of baptismal preparation as it was practiced at the time. It even seems that Philip's conduct as far as baptism was concerned was not always exemplary. The case of Simon the Magician (Acts 8:9-25) shows that he tended to proceed more hastily than he should. One may wonder if his attachment to the community of Caesarea (Acts 21:8-9), which ended his admirable itinerant charism (while St. Paul was beginning his), was not motivated by the necessity to give him some balance and to restrict him by an established authority.

[6]Augustine, *De fide et op.*, 8,13; FC 27, p. 235.

[7]Cf. below, pp. 19-20.

[8]A. Turck. "Aux origines du catéchuménat," in *Revue des sciences philosophiques et théologiques*, 48 (1964), pp. 20-31.

[9]Cf. Acts 16:30; 22:8-10; and Lk 3:10.

[10]Cf. the table in Dujarier, *Parrainage des adultes*, pp. 391-3.

[11]P. Benoit, "Qumrân et le Nouveau Testament," *New Testament Studies*, 7, 1961, pp. 276-96. The influence of the baptismal practices of Essenism and Judaism is argued by A. Jaubert: "Acts mention that a great number of the priests were obedient to the faith (Acts 6:7). . . . It seems reasonable to admit that [these priests] came from circles that opposed the official orientations and had an affinity with John the Baptist. Thus the ancient Christian community could receive little by little the influx of a long sacerdotal tradition, which was valuable for its liturgical organization." *Les Premiers Chrétiens*, Paris, 1967. Cf. J. Thomas, *Le Mouvement baptiste en Palestine et Syrie (150 av. J.-C.—300 ap. J.-C.)*, unpublished dissertation, Leuven, 1935.

[12]Josephus, *The Jewish War, The Loeb Classical Library* 203, translated by H. St. J. Thackery, London, William Heinemann, 1967, p. 375 (Bk II §§137-138).

28

[13]Dujarier, *Parrainage des adultes,* pp. 99-111.

[14]*Règle* 5, 13-14; tr. J. Carmignac, *Les Textes de Qumrân,* vol. 1, Paris, 1969.

[15]Dujarier, *Parrainage des adultes,* pp. 73-97.

[16]See also Gerim I, in Dujarier, op. cit., p. 82. Cf. Lk 7,1-10.

[17]See also Gerim I, in Dujarier, op. cit., p. 89.

[18]B. Bagatti, *L'Eglise de la Circoncision,* Jerusalem, 1965, pp. 195-206. To the witnesses mentioned by Bagatti, I would add Justin, "Dialogue with Tryphon," 122.5 and the many others cited by Lampe in *A Patristic Greek Lexicon,* p. 1171.

The Structuring of the
Catechumenate
(Second-Third Centuries)

Up until 313, the Church had to survive under very difficult circumstances. Numerically, it had relatively few adherents; socially, its members were immersed in a pagan world; politically, it had no rights and was persecuted. But the difficulty of this situation made permanent demands that were ultimately the source of pastoral strength. The Church exercised its apostolate in an eminently missionary context. It is precisely during this period that the catechumenate became structured and took on its most authentic form.[1]

I shall trace the major stages of this development through some typical examples. But first, let us examine the spirit that guided this pastoral effort.

An Abiding Concern for Pastoral Authenticity

WE have already stressed the concern the ministers of baptism had from the very beginning for the sincerity of the conversion of the candidates. This same concern for authenticity would guide the missionary Church in its maternal function during the second and third centuries. It is essential that one never forget that the salvific power of Christ cannot work where, because of a lack of faith, the circumstances are not favorable (Mt 13:58). In other words, the sacrament cannot be given to a subject who is not properly disposed or whose faith has not really transformed his or her life.

Let us consider two typical witnesses among those that emphasize the necessity of a certain period of time to consolidate the conversion and to form the convert.

In North Africa

For Tertullian, baptism is the "seal of the faith,"[2] of a faith that had to be awakened and deepened beforehand. The initiation is to be conceived as the one entrance into the one faith but by successive stages. With regard to the faith, the catechumenal journey is expressed in three actions: assent to the faith, entrance into the faith, and sealing of the faith. Reciprocally, baptism is realized progressively from the initial fear of God to the sacramental experience of

God through a healthy and penitent faith. This is what Tertullian said to the catechumens of Carthage who were delaying their conversion because of a "presumptuous confidence in baptism":

> The Lord will begin by verifying the quality of the penitence before granting us a reward as magnificent as eternal life.—9. Who would dare, indeed, grant you, whose penitence is so uncertain, sprinkling with whatever kind of water?—12. Some think that God is obliged to grant, even to the unworthy, what he has promised: they transform his generosity into servitude.—16. This baptismal bath is the seal of the faith, but this faith is begun in the sincerity of penitence and is therein guaranteed.—17. We are not washed to end our sins, but because we have ended them, we have already been bathed in our hearts; this is in fact the first baptism of the hearer [of the Word]. From then on, a perfect fear that the Lord will recognize, a healthy faith and a conscience that has embraced penitence once and for all.—22. Whom would you judge to be the more worthy, if not the best amended, and who is the best amended, if not the one who has the greatest fear of God and who, on this account, has truly repented?[3]

The practice of the "officials" must match this teaching, the officials whose role it is to discern the sincerity of the candidates in order to avoid being circumvented by those who would approach under false pretenses.

> Let those whose function it is know that

baptism may not be granted lightly. "Give to anyone who asks of you" [Lk 6:30] envisages alms in the strict sense. [For baptism], you must instead take into account this [word]: "Do not give to dogs what is holy and do not throw your pearls before swine" [Mt 7:6] and: "Do not lay on hands hastily and do not be an accomplice to another man's sins" [I Tim 5:22].[4]

In Palestine

The homilies Origen preached around 240 at Caesarea echo the pastoral principles enunciated by Tertullian. Baptism is indeed a gift from God but a gift that, to be efficacious, presupposes a real change of life on the part of the recipient, a transformation of morals in the light of the law of Christ.

> You who desire to receive baptism and to merit the grace of the Spirit, you must first be purified from the law: you must first, upon hearing the Word of God, root out your habitual vices and allay your barbaric customs so that, having been clothed in meekness and humility, you will be able to receive the Holy Spirit.[5]

> Come, catechumens, do penance to receive the baptism in remission of sins. He receives baptism for the remission of sins who ceases to sin. If, however, someone comes to baptism while continuing to sin, for him, there is no remission of sins. This is why, I beg of you, do not come to baptism without examining it closely and without profound consideration, and show first of all

> "the worthy fruit of penance" [Lk 3:8]. Spend a certain amount of time in good conduct and keep yourselves free of all vice and of all [kinds of] grossness: thus, you will obtain the remission of sins when you begin, you also, to despise your sins.[6]

We shall see further on how these demands were realized. But let us dwell here for a moment on the categorical affirmation, both in the East and in the West, of the necessity of a preparatory period for baptism that permits the candidate effectively to alter his or her life in function of the new faith so that the reception of the sacrament not be a mockery.

> Heed well, catechumens, listen and profit from what I say in order to prepare yourselves while you are not yet baptized. Come to the fountain, be washed for salvation; do not be content with being washed, like some who have been content and who have not been washed for salvation, who have received the water and not the Holy Spirit, while those who have been washed for salvation receive the water and the Holy Spirit together.[7]

It is with this theological vision of an essential bond uniting faith and sacrament that I shall now turn to the evolution of the catechumenal ministry in the second and third centuries in the various Churches of the Mediterranean world.

In Rome ca. 150

It was around the year 180 that what we have come to call the "catechumenate" was born.[8] In reality, it was less an institution than a way of doing things, a usage that spread rather rapidly and was subsequently recognized by the Church as the most suitable means to prepare converts for baptism.

At the end of the first century in Syria, according to the *Didache*, Christian initiation already presupposed a certain period of catechetical instructions.[9] Around the year 140 in Rome—the technical term "catechumen" was not yet being used—the "Shepherd" of Hermas witnesses to the existence of a true journey by those preparing for the sacraments. In his third vision Hermas sees the Church as a tower under construction "that is being built on the waters with brilliant squared stones." He notes that some stones "fell near the water and do not succeed in rolling in, in spite of their desire." These stones, he is told, represent

> those who have heard the word of God and who want to be baptized in the name of the Lord. Only, when they remember the sanctity that the truth demands, they change their minds and turn again to their evil passions.[10]

We certainly have here a trace of the baptismal requirements the Church clearly placed on the "hearers of the word," who are the candidates. If some of them changed their minds, it was because there was a probationary delay before baptism and that it was necessary to give evidence of conversion.

The organization of the catechumenate that we meet in Hippolytus around 215 did not appear suddenly: it was the fruit of a pastoral effort that took shape throughout the second century. We have another witness in the First Apology of Justin of this slow maturation, which is already reflected in the work of Hermas. I cite the most important passage. Even though he only describes the baptismal initiation as such (with its three elements: final communal liturgical preparation, baptism, eucharist), he clearly alludes to preliminary instructions, the characteristics of which we shall try to specify.

> 61. I will also relate the manner in which we dedicated ourselves to God when we had been made new through Christ; lest, if we omit this, we seem to be unfair in the explanation we are making. As many are persuaded and believe that what we teach and say is true, and undertake to be able to live accordingly, are instructed to pray and to entreat God with fasting, for the remission of their sins that are past, we praying and fasting with them. Then they are brought by us where there is water, and are regenerated in the same manner in which we were ourselves regenerated. For, in the name of God, the Father and Lord of the universe, and of our Saviour Jesus Christ, and of the Holy Spirit, they then receive the washing with water.

> 65. But we, after we have thus washed him who has been convinced and has assented to our teaching, bring him to the place where

those who are called brethren are assembled, in order that we may offer hearty prayers in common for ourselves and for the baptized [illuminated] person, and for all others in every place, that we may be counted worthy, now that we have learned the truth, by our works also to be found good citizens and keepers of the commandments, so that we may be saved with an everlasting salvation.

66. This food is called among us Εὐχαριστία of which no one is allowed to partake but the man who believes that the things which we teach are true, and who has been washed with the washing that is for the remission of sins, and unto regeneration, and who is so living as Christ has enjoined.[11]

The Preliminary Evangelization

In this epoch, apostolic labor was not reserved to a few specialists. Each individual Christian was involved in leading his neighbors to the faith. Justin gives us an example:

A certain woman lived with an intemperate husband; she herself, too, having formerly been intemperate. But when she came to the knowledge of the teachings of Christ she became sober-minded, and endeavoured to persuade her husband likewise to be temperate, citing the teaching of Christ, and assuring him that there shall be punishment in eternal fire inflicted upon those who do not live temperately and conformably to right reason.[12]

The proclamation of the Good News was not the privilege of priests or scholars. It was a mission that all Christians, even the least educated, were determined to accomplish according to their own grace and opportunity.

> Among us these things can be heard and learned from persons who do not even know the forms of the letters, who are uneducated and barbarous in speech, though wise and believing in mind; some, indeed even maimed and deprived of eyesight.[13]

Evangelization was thus accomplished flexibly and spontaneously, but it still had to be serious and the instructions themselves thorough. This is why admission to baptism was subject to quite specific requirements to which I shall return later. Some Christians dedicated themselves more particularly to the task of awakening faith and of teaching and opened "schools" as did philosophers of this period. These were private initiatives and were not institutionalized.[14] The hierarchical Church had not yet assumed the direct responsibility for the teaching given in them. But the fact is clear: the laity themselves carefully ensured the evangelization and instruction of converts.

Criteria for Access to Baptism

Admission to baptism, therefore, represented the issue of a rather long preparation. It was subject to three, already very precise, requirements:

First, sorrow for sins, since baptism is "for the remission of sins."[15] Justin insisted on this point and cited the famous text of Isaiah 1:16-20, "cease to do evil, learn to do good," which the fathers often commented upon in the course of their baptismal catechesis.[16]

Second, faith in the Church as the teacher of truth: everything it teaches, everything it says must be welcomed as the truth.[17] This requirement obviously presupposes thorough preliminary instruction.

Finally, transformation of life: one has to "undertake to be able to live accordingly."[18] How could one be able to do this unless there had been a sufficient period, parallel to the instructions, to bring about a true moral conversion? Whether it concerned the eucharist or baptism, the sacrament was only granted to those who live "as Christ has enjoined."[19]

The period of formation, as flexible as it was during this period, was thus submitted to the discernment of the Church, which judged the aptitude of the candidates on the basis of these fundamental criteria.

But baptism was still not granted immediately. The administration of the sacrament was preceded by a certain amount of time that can be called the "baptismal period."

The Baptismal Period

Before baptism, there were a few days of liturgical preparation. This was already the custom in Syria at the end of the first century. The *Didache* states:

> . . . before the baptism, let the one who baptizes and the one to be baptized fast, and any others who are able to do so. And you shall require the person being baptized to fast for one or two days.[20]

In Justin's time, many of the faithful joined the

future neophytes and prayed and fasted with them[21] and actively initiated them into the community worship. Finally, they accompanied them from the place of baptism and introduced them into the larger community of the "brothers" to celebrate together the eucharist.[22]

The witness of Justin thus manifests the essential aspects of stages and catechumenal requirements. In the course of the following decades, these stages and requirements were codified more and more strictly.

In Egypt ca. 190-200

AT the end of the second century in Egypt, there was not any apparent codification of the catechumenate. But there were customs and a vocabulary that manifest the existence of serious catechumenal formation.

According to Eusebius of Caesarea, Pantaenus had founded a "school of catechesis" in Alexandria and Clement succeeded him as the head around 190. This has been questioned by some scholars, but it seems that the information furnished by Eusebius is exact.[23] In any event, the works of Clement witness unambiguously to the use of the word "catechumen" and the practice of a real catechumenal discipline. There are many texts that indicate this. Here are some that mutually clarify each other.

First, from the side of the catechists, we see that a very great intellectual effort was made to sustain the values of Greek philosophy:

> Erudition recommends the master who presents the principal dogmas, it helps to persuade the listeners, it rouses admiration of the catechumens and forms them to the Truth.[24]
>
> Most of those who inscribe their name, it seems, such as the companions of Ulysses, are vulgar followers of the Word. . . . But he who welcomes what is useful in [Hellenic studies] for the instruction of the catechumens ought not to abstain from [using] his erudition, but should have it contribute as much as possible to help his listeners.[25]

We note that this instruction envisaged increasing

the faith of those preparing for baptism:

> Catechesis leads progressively to the faith;
> the faith, at the moment of baptism, receives
> the instruction of the Holy Spirit.[26]
> The "beings of flesh"—one can say that they
> are the new catechumens, still "little ones" in
> Christ. The Apostle indeed gave the name of
> "spirituals" to those who already have the
> faith by the Holy Spirit, while he calls "car-
> nal" the newly catechized who have yet to
> receive the purfication [of baptism].[27]

This education was not purely intellectual. Note
where the distinction is made between the baptized
and those preparing for baptism: the catechumens
"want" to live in a Christian manner while the faithful,
because of the sacrament, have also received the
"power" to do so. There is no doubt that the converts
were not admitted to the sacrament until they were
examined on the seriousness of the conversion:

> For some, there is already, with the will, the
> power to do, when they have developed it by
> exercise and have purified themselves; oth-
> ers, even though they are not yet able,
> possess at least the desire. . . . And definite-
> ly, one does not judge the acts only according
> to their execution, but one judges them also
> according to the deliberate intention of each:
> Was the choice made lightly? Have the faults
> been repented of? Is he aware of his failures?
> And has he recognized them?[28]

There is every indication that this vital conversion
required formation over a certain period of time.
Clement tells us that it lasted at least three years after
inscription.[29]

[The Law] does not allow imperfect fruit to be harvested from imperfect trees, but [it desires] that after three years the first fruits of the harvest be dedicated in the fourth year to God, when the tree has reached its perfection. This agricultural image can be a lesson: it teaches us the necessity of pruning the excrescences of faults and this vain vegetation of thought that grows at the same time as the natural fruits until the new structure of the faith attains its perfect size and solidity. It is indeed in the fourth year—since time is also necessary for solid catechumenal formation—that the tetrad of virtues is consecrated to God, the third stage already touching on the fourth that is the house of the Lord.[30]

Thus, we may conclude with A. Méhat that the works of Clement reveal the existence of a catechumenate in Alexandria around the year 200. They clearly affirm that there were catechumens who inscribed their names and received instruction and formation over a number of years with a view to baptism. Even though the structure of the school of catechesis was very flexible, and even though pagans and neophytes mixed with the catechumens to listen to this teaching, one thing is certain: there was a group of converts who followed a special course of formation before being admitted to the sacraments of initiation.

It is inconceivable that terms as specialized as "catechesis" and "catechumens" were employed by Clement in senses entirely different than they had for Origen a generation later, than they had for Tertullian at almost the same period.[31]

In North Africa ca. 200-210

WHILE Clement was teaching and writing in Egypt, the Christian communities of North Africa were living the same catechumenal reality and using the same vocabulary. Let it suffice here to mention the "Passion of SS. Perpetua and Felicity." The events recounted occurred in 202-203. In the very first lines, the narrative confronts us with a group of catechumens arrested for their faith:

> The young catechumens were arrested: Revocatus and Felicity, her slave companion, Saturninus and Secundulus. With them, Vibia Perpetua, of noble birth, well-educated, married and matron, still having her father, mother, and two brothers, one of whom was a catechumen.[32]

To discern the traces of the appearance of the catechumenate, one must be attentive to various terms that designate the converts on the road to baptism. The word "catechumen" was used the most, but it is neither the first nor the only term that was used. We have already met "proselyte of Christ." There are many others.

In addition to "catechumen," which was transcribed from the Greek and which Tertullian often used, we also find—as already in Clement and soon in Cyprian—the well-known term "auditor" *(audiens, auditor)*. Less often cited, but of particular interest, is the term "recruit" *(tiro)* which is used in opposition to "soldier" *(miles)*. These two appellations correspond exactly to the distinction Tertullian makes between the "catechumens" and the "faithful" when he criticizes the Marcionites:

> It is uncertain who is a catechumen and who is a baptized believer: they all alike reproach, they all alike hear, they all alike pray—even heathens, if any should have chanced to enter. They will "throw that which is holy to dogs and pearls (albeit false ones) to swine." . . .The catechumens are certainly initiated before being instructed.[33]

In his treatise on penitence, Tertullian calls catechumens "novices" *(noviciol)* [34] and he speaks in their regard of a "military novitiate" *(tirocinia*, in the plural, which corresponds to what are called *"les classes"* in the French army[35]). These military expressions, which clearly distinguish between the young recruit who is in basic training and the soldier who has taken his oath and has been branded, are also found in Commodian, who is thought to have been an African who lived in the third century. In his "Instructions," there is an address "to the catechumens" where a clear equivalence is established between *tiro* and catechumen:

> Believers in Christ who have abandoned the idols, all,
> I counsel you, in a few words, for your salvation.
> If, in the beginning, you were living in error, dedicate yourself to Christ from now on, abandon all things
> and, since you know God, be a good recruit, [become] a tested soldier,
> and let your virginal modesty live in the Lamb.

> Let the spirit of the righteous remain alert:
> beware of sinning as before;
> baptism removes only the original stain.
> If any catechumen comes to sin,
> he is struck with a penalty,
> marked by a penalty, you will be able to live
> [in Christ]
> but not without damage.
> Above all, always avoid grave faults.[36]

Thus it is certain that, in the years 200-210, there existed in Carthage as in Alexandria a period of catechumenal formation to which all those who aspired to baptism were subject. They were not admitted to sacramental initiation unless the Church, through the agency of those responsible, observed the authenticity of their conversion.[37]

At the end of their catechumenate, those who were thus admitted formed the group of "those entering baptism" *(ingressuri baptismum)*. These were the "blessed" *(benedicti)*. They spent a certain period— probably a week[38]—in prayer, vigils, and fasting:

> Those who are going to enter baptism must invoke God by fervent prayers, fastings, kneelings, and vigils. They also prepare themselves by the confession of all their past sins. . . . By afflicting the flesh and the spirit, we provide satisfaction for sin and protect ourselves in advance against the temptation to come. . . .
>
> You, therefore, the blessed, you for whom God's grace awaits, you who shall go up to the most holy bath of the new birth, you who, for the first time, shall hold out your hands next to a Mother and with brothers, ask the

> Father, ask the Lord, as a special gift of his grace, for the abundance of his charisms.[39]

Baptism itself could take place any time but Easter was preferred "when the Passion of the Lord is consummated in which we are baptized." It could also be conferred during Pentecost which, at that time, was not a particular feast fifty days after Easter, but the feast of the fifty days of the Paschal Season: "the time when the grace of the Holy Spirit was communicated to the disciples and that provides a glimpse of their hope in the return of the Lord."[40]

As for the way in which baptism itself was administered, Tertullian has only left us a few indications.[41] I cite the most explicit passage from his treatise, "The Chaplet":

> When we are about to enter the water, and, as a matter of fact, even a short while before, we declare in the presence of the congregation before the bishop that we renounce the Devil, his pomps, and his angels. After that, we are immersed in the water three times, making a somewhat fuller pledge than the Lord has prescribed in the Gospel. After this, having stepped forth from the font, we are given a taste of a mixture of milk and honey and from that day, for a whole week, we forego our daily bath.[42]

In Rome ca. 215

THE *Apostolic Tradition* of Hippolytus shows that the catechumenal stages were not empty words at the beginning of the third century in Rome. Not only was the catechumenate a long period of formation—it usually lasted three years—but it was also situated between two very thorough examinations for admission. Of course, this is not to be taken in an academic sense, but rather as an indication of the importance of the questions posed at these critical moments and of the guarantees they elicited in response.

Entry into the Catechumenate

Admission to the catechumenate was already selective, and some candidates were refused because of the impurity of their motives. Those whom we now call sponsors, i.e. the Christians who evangelized these postulants and who accompanied them to the Church, had to witness to their aptitude to become catechumens. Did they have enough faith to "hear the word" during catechesis? Even the opinion of Christian employers was asked when their employees were involved.

> Those who come forward the first time to hear the word shall first be brought to the teachers at the house before all the people come in. And let them be examined as to the reason why they have come forward to the faith. And those who bring them shall bear

witness for them whether they are able to
hear. Let their life and manner of living be
enquired into, whether he has a wife and
whether he is a slave or free. If he be the
slave of a believer and his master permit him,
let him hear. If his master does not bear
witness to him, let him be rejected. If his
master be a heathen, let him be taught "to
please his master" that there be no scandal.[43]

Then the accepted candidates were informed of the
basic requirements of the Christian life:

If a man have a wife or a woman a husband,
let them be taught the man to be contented
with his wife and the woman to be contented
with her husband. A man who is unmarried
let him be taught not to commit fornication
but either to marry lawfully or to abide
steadfast.

But if there be one who has a devil, let him
not hear the word from the teacher until he
be cleansed.

The postulants were also required to abandon their
profession if it was contrary to Christian morals, i.e.
one that led to the commission of one of the three
major sins: idolatry, homicide, or impurity:

They shall enquire about the crafts and
occupations of those who are brought for
instruction. If a man be a pander who sup-
ports harlots either let him desist or let him
be rejected. If a man be a sculptor or a
painter, he shall be taught not to make idols.
If he will not desist, let him be rejected. If a
man be an actor or one who makes shows in

the theatre, either let him desist or let him be rejected. If a man teach children worldly knowledge, it is indeed well if he desist. But if he has no other trade by which to live, let him have forgiveness. A charioteer likewise or one who takes part in the games or who goes to the games, either let him desist or let him be rejected. A man who is a gladiator or a trainer of gladiators or a huntsman in the arena or one concerned with wild-beast shows or a public official who is concerned with gladiatorial shows either let him desist or let him be rejected. If a man be a priest of idols or a keeper of idols either let him desist or let him be rejected. A soldier who is in authority must be told not to execute men; if he should be ordered to do it, he shall not do it. He must be told not to take the military oath. If he will not agree, let him be rejected. A military governor or a magistrate of a city who wears the purple, either let him desist or let him be rejected. If a catechumen or a baptised Christian wishes to become a soldier, let him be cast out. For he has despised God. A harlot or a sodomite or one who has castrated himself or one who does things which may not be spoken of, let them be rejected for they are defiled. A magician shall not even be brought for consideration. A charmer or an astrologer or an interpreter of dreams or a mountebank or a clipper of fringes of clothes or a maker of amulets, let them desist or let them be rejected. If a man's concubine be a slave, let her hear on condition that she have reared her children, and if she consorts with him alone. But if not let her be rejected. If a man have a concubine, let him desist and marry legally; and if he will not, let him be rejected.

If we have omitted anything, decide ye as is fit; for we all have the Spirit of God.[44]

The Catechesis

Catechesis was provided by teachers, clerical or lay. In principle, it lasted for three years:

> Let a catechumen be instructed for three years. But if a man be earnest and persevere well in the matter, let him be received, because it is not the time that is judged, but the conduct.
>
> Each time the teacher finishes his instruction let the catechumens pray by themselves apart from the faithful. And let the women stand in the assembly by themselves apart from the men, both the baptised women and the women catechumens.
>
> But after the prayer is finished the catechumens shall not give the kiss of peace for their kiss is not yet pure. . . .
>
> After the prayer of the catechumens let the teacher lay hands upon them and pray and dismiss them. Whether the teacher be an ecclesiastic or a layman let him do the same.[45]

The catechesis was given during the community celebration, which normally took place in the morning before work. The catechumens thus do not seem to have been placed in a special group: they were already in the Church, even though they were not yet full members. They participated in the liturgy of the word at the same time as the faithful,[46] but they were assigned a special place at the meeting and did not give the kiss of peace.[47]

At the end of this common liturgy, the catechist said a special prayer for the catechumens. The imposition of hands that preceded it was probably a gesture of exorcism.[48]

Admission to Baptism

Admission to baptism called for another examination. The sponsors again had to give witness but, this time, they testified to the conduct of the catechumens during the instruction period. Those who were judged suitable became the "chosen" and could then hear the Gospel, that is, be admitted to the baptismal liturgy.

> And when they are chosen who are set apart to receive baptism let their life be examined, whether they lived piously while catechumens, whether "they honoured the widows," whether they visited the sick, whether they have fulfilled every good work.
>
> If those who bring them bear witness to them that they have done thus, then let them hear the gospel.[49]

Thus began the baptismal period, which, as we have seen in Tertullian, probably lasted for a week.[50] Each day the chosen ones were exorcised by an imposition of hands. Then a more solemn exorcism was administered by the bishop.

> Moreover, from the day they are chosen, let a hand be laid on them and let them be

exorcised daily. And when the day draws near on which they are to be baptised, let the bishop himself exorcise each one of them, that he may be certain that he is purified.

But if there is one who is not purified let him be put on one side because he did not hear the word of instruction with faith. For the evil and strange spirit remained with him.

And let those who are to be baptised be instructed to wash and cleanse themselves on the fifth day of the week. And if any woman be menstruous she shall be put aside and be baptised another day.

Those who are to receive baptism shall fast on the Friday and on the Saturday. And on the Saturday the bishop shall assemble those who are to be baptised in one place, and shall bid them all to pray and bow the knee.

And laying his hand on them he shall exorcise every evil spirit to flee away from them and never to return to them henceforward. And when he has finished exorcising, let him breathe on their faces and seal their foreheads and ears and noses and then let him raise them up.

And they shall spend all the night in vigil, reading the scriptures to them and instructing them.

Moreover those who are to be baptised shall not bring any other vessel, save that which each will bring with him for the eucharist. For it is right for every one to bring his oblation then.[51]

After having described the initiation celebration,[52] Hippolytus adds a very significant phrase. He stresses that baptism and the eucharist, far from being a terminus, are a beginning, the beginning of a life in which one must ceaselessly grow:

> And when these things have been accomplished, let each one be zealous to perform good works and to please God, living righteously, devoting himself to the Church, performing the things which he has learnt, advancing in the service of God.[53]

A catechumenal discipline as strict as that presented by the *Apostolic Tradition* is not unique for this period. We have seen that its seed was present in the apostolic period and that it grew little by little during the second century. And we have seen that the same requirements were imposed around the year 200 in the churches of Alexandria and Carthage. This discipline was affirmed in the following decades, especially in the eastern portion of the Mediterranean world.

In Egypt and Palestine
ca. 230-240

THE best witnesses to the vitality of the catechumenal stages during the first half of the third century in Egypt and Palestine are provided by the great catechist Origen. This astonishingly dynamic man never ceased to concern himself with the seriousness of baptismal formation. In the expanding Church of his time, it hurt him to see numbers threatening to submerge quality, and he struggled for the purity of the Christian life as it was during the second century. Already then he spoke words that apply to us today:

> If we judge things according to the truth…, we have to recognize that we are not faithful. They were truly faithful then when martyrdom struck from the birth [of the Church]. . ., when the catechumens were catechized in the midst of martyrs and of the death of Christians who confessed the truth to the end, when these catechumens, surmounting these trials, attach themselves without fear to the living God . . . . Then the faithful were fewer, certainly, but they were truly faithful, advancing by the harsh and narrow way that leads to life.[54]

With his permanent concern to maintain an authentic Christianity, Origen always strove for a catechumenate of quality. Let us first see how he conceived this institution, and then we shall be able to specify the two great stages: evangelization and catechesis.

The Catechumenate by Stages

Origen often compared baptismal preparation to the biblical event of the Exodus. Though he considered the crossing of the desert by the Hebrew people as an image of the Christian life leading from baptism to entrance into heaven, he also considered this event as an image of the catechumenal journey extending from conversion (departure from Egypt) and the entrance into the catechumenate (crossing of the Red Sea) to baptism (crossing the River Jordan), which marks the entry into the Kingdom of Christ (the Promised Land). Here is how he addresses the catechumens:

> When you abandon the darkness of idolatry and when you desire to arrive at the knowledge of the divine law, then begin your departure from Egypt. When you have been accepted into the crowd of the catechumens and when you have begun to obey the commandments of the Church, you have crossed the Red Sea. In the halts in the desert, each day, you apply yourself to listening to the law of God and to contemplate the visage of Moses which discloses the glory of the Lord. But when you arrive at the spiritual spring of baptism and when in the presence of the sacerdotal and levitical order you will be initiated into these venerable and sublime mysteries that are only known by those who have the right to know them; then, having crossed the Jordan, thanks to the ministry of the priests, you will enter in the land of the promise, this land where Jesus, after Moses, takes you in charge and becomes the guide for your new path.[55]

When, from the darkness of error, you are led to the light of knowledge, when, from a terrestial life, you are converted to the beginnings of the spiritual life, you leave Egypt and you enter into the desert, that is into a kind of life in which, in the midst of silence and calm, you practice the divine laws and you are impregnated with the celestial oracles. Then, when you have undergone their formation and direction, after having crossed the Jordan, you hasten to the Promised Land, that is when, by the grace of baptism, you arrive at the evangelical precepts.[56]

These texts are witness of primary importance to the existence of catechumenal stages. In addition, they show the advantage of using expressive biblical images, which are easy to explain in a vivid manner to catechumens.

Evangelization

In the journey toward baptism, the catechumenate is not the first step. It follows a period of search and discovery that is too often forgotten. This is the time of evangelization, a period during which, after interest has been aroused in Christ or Christianity, direct contact is made with individual Christians.

This is the period when the Good News is proclaimed and awakens a global act of faith in the Christian mystery; it is the period of the first conversion to Christ that implies a decision to transform one's life, without which none would succeed in being admitted to the catechumenate.

Who does this evangelization? Those who continue the itinerant mission of the apostles:

> . . . as far as they are able Christians leave no stone unturned to spread the faith in all parts of the world. Some, in fact, have done the work of going round not only cities but even villages and country cottages to make others also pious toward God.[57]

The missionary task was a concern of the entire Church. In addition to those permanently engaged in evangelization, there was the mass of Christians who announced the Good News to those around them. They did this spontaneously in their daily lives, not as a tactic, but naturally, on the basis of the relationships they had with their relatives, friends, and co-workers, each according to his charism.

Origen reports how a pagan, Celsus, described the evangelical activity of the laity (ca. 180):

> In private houses also we see wool-workers, cobblers, laundry-workers, and the most illiterate and bucolic yokels, who would not dare to say anything at all in front of their elders and more intelligent masters. But whenever they get hold of children in private and some stupid women with them, they let out some astounding statements. . . . they alone, they say, know the right way to live . . . . if they like, they should leave father and their schoolmasters, and go along with the women and little children who are their playfellows to the wooldresser's shop, or to the cobbler's or the washerwoman's shop, that they may learn perfection. And by saying this they persuade them.[58]

What was the content of this first proclamation, this

kerygma? It seems that it concerned the problem of the Living God and idolatry: God the Creator, the one God who loves man, who can be recognized in one's life and in history. In opposition to the religious authorities of paganism, they presented Jesus, sent by God, who took on our condition until death to open for us a transformed and infinite life. So the faith was awakened among those who were drawn by the manner of life of the Christians and who had begun to welcome Christ. This is how Origen answers Celsus, although the following passage probably concerns the first catechesis as well as chance conversations in shops or homes:

> We clearly show the sacred character of our origin, and do not conceal it, as Celsus thinks, since even in people only just converted we inculcate a scorn of idols and all images, and in addition to this raise their thoughts from serving created things in the place of God and lift them up to the Creator of the universe. We prove clearly that he was the one prophesied by quoting both from the prophecies about him (and there are many of them), and from the gospels and the utterances of the apostles, which are carefully explained by those who are able to understand them intelligently.[59]

It is always the same common theme that we already find germinally in I Thessalonians 1:9-10: rejection of idols and recognition of the one Creator and faith in Christ. This is accompanied by an account of the excellence and purity of Christianity and terminates in an explicit appeal to receive the Kingdom.[60]

Admission to the Catechumenate

Entrance to the catechumenate was not granted immediately. First, there had to be a certain time of formation and probation, what we might call a postulancy. The postulant would only be "admitted to the number of the catechumens" after he or she had accepted the kerygma, that is, after having made an act of faith and manifested conversion by beginning to change his or her life. Catechesis was not open to just anybody:

> . . . philosophers who converse in public do not select their hearers, but anyone interested stops to listen. But as far as they can, Christians previously examine the souls of those who want to hear them, and test them individually beforehand; when before entering the community the hearers seem to have devoted themselves sufficiently to the desire to live a good life, then they introduce them.[61]

Here again is the examination of admission to the catechumenate that was mentioned by Hippolytus. In addition to affirming the practice, Origen also gives us information on the preliminary evangelization of which the *Apostolic Tradition* does not speak. The first instructions, according to Origen, concerned mainly the awakening of faith, and it was done in homes and workshops and not in a formal way. What we would today call, very inexactly, the "precatechumenate" was then living contact with Christians. It was evangelical witness, with the Christians playing more the role of sponsors than of teachers. What was involved was the radiation of a Christian community inserted in the larger human community, not intellectual instruction by an institutional staff.

Hippolytus speaks only of the examination of admission to the catechumenate and does not describe the accompanying liturgical rite that changed a postulant into a catechumen. In a passage in his "Exhortation to Martyrdom," Origen possibly alludes to this rite. When writing to Christians who were frightened at the prospect of the supreme sacrifice, he reminded them of the commitment they had made on the specific occasion of beginning catechesis. If this commitment had not been made, the catechist would have had nothing more to do with them, as Origen shows in this fictitious dialogue:

> At the beginning when you were to be instructed in the Christian faith it would have been reasonable to say to you: "If you do not wish to serve the Lord, choose you this day whom you will serve, whether the gods of your fathers on the far side of the river or the gods of the Amorites, among whom you inhabit the land." And the catechist might have said to you: "As for me and my house, we will serve the Lord, for he is holy." But now it is not possible to say this to you. For at that time you said: "God forbid that we should forsake the Lord and serve other gods. The Lord our God, he is God, who brought us and our fathers up out of Egypt and kept us in all the way in which we journeyed." Moreover, in the agreements concerning religion you long ago made this reply to your instructors: "We will serve the Lord, for he is our God."[62]

Such a text—and this one seems to be unknown to many historians of the catechumenate—gives a good idea of what could have been the decision of faith demanded of the postulant before admission to catechesis. Note that these are the same words as those used in the dialogue of Joshua with the Hebrews at the sealing of the covenant at Shechem (Jos. 24:14-24). These are decisive covenant formulas, and those who enter the covenant are themselves witnesses of their commitment (Jos. 22:22,27). Thus the commencement of catechesis presupposes an event analogous to the sealing of the covenant at Shechem. This is why it is appropriate to apply this text to catechumens, and the way in which Origen teaches them to read their experience in the very word of God is admirable.

Although Origen clearly states that a commitment was made at the start of catechesis, we do not know its form. Was there a liturgical rite, a specific meeting? Probably. But Origen's text does not warrant such an affirmation since it is clear that the words are placed by Origen in the mouths of the catechist and the catechumens and were not spoken as such. Rather, their purpose is to convey the value and the validity of the commitment.

The Catechumenal Period

The catechumenate was a period of formation in the Christian faith and morals. Origen states that there were two groups of catechumens:

> They privately appoint one class consisting of recent beginners who are receiving elementary instruction and have not yet received the sign that they have been purified, and an-

other class of those who, as far as they are able, make it their set purpose to desire nothing other than those things of which Christians approve.[63]

The first group consisted of the catechumens in the strict sense of the word; the second were the "chosen ones," who had virtually finished their formation. They were chosen by the Church as being suitable for baptism because it saw that they could live as Christians, not simply because they want to. It is of them that Origen writes further on:

> But when some of those who have been thus encouraged make progress and show that they have been purified by the Logos, and do all in their power to live better lives, then we call them to our mysteries.[64]

As in Rome, the two examinations for admission to the catechumenate and to baptism were thus applied very seriously and both involved a transformation of life. Moreover, it was not the candidate himself who judged his own aptitude but the members of the Church who were designated for this function and whose judgment was based on the testimony of the Christians who evangelized him. This is very clear for the admission to the stages of the catechumenate:

> Among the latter class some are appointed to inquire into the lives and conduct of those who want to join the community in order that they may prevent those who indulge in secret sins from coming to their common gathering; those who do not do this they whole-heartedly receive, and make them better every day.[65]

In Syria and Palestine ca. 250

THE practice of catechumenal stages that we have noted in all the countries of the Mediterranean world at the beginning of the third century was not an isolated idea of a few creative catechists. It was the normal way of doing things and it developed spontaneously everywhere. The Church recognized its authenticity and necessity. Further proof of this is given by a canonico-liturgical document written in Syria between 230 and 250, the *Didascalia of the Apostles.*

The Didascalia

Written by a bishop, this work is concerned primarily with the structuring of the penitential discipline. It does this on the basis of the catechumenal discipline. Is not penitence, as Origen stressed, a kind of repeat of baptism and, as such, does it not require a new probation in stages? Thus the *Didascalia* enables us to describe the stages of the catechumenate as the Church applied them in Syria around 250.[66]

Evangelization was the work of the laity who converted their friends, who "familiarized" them in order to introduce them into the Church "confirmed and believing."[67]

Admission to the catechumenate supposes an authentic conversion:

> We do not refuse salvation even to the heathen if they repent and renounce and remove themselves from error . . . when they wish and promise to repent and say, "We

believe," we receive them into the congregation that they may hear the Word, but we do
not communicate with them until they receive the seal and are confirmed.[68]

The catechumenate would then be this time of
formation when the candidates "hear the Word" and
show the worthy fruits of penitence until the day
when they would be judged fit to enter into the
baptismal period.

The Apocryphal Acts of the Apostles

In addition to the *Didascalia,* which reflects the
discipline the hierarchy wished to impose, we have
many popular writings that claim to give the lives of
the apostles. These edifying tales are of great interest
to us since they occasionally provide information on
the catechumenal practice of the first half of the third
century and some of them even for the end of the
second century.

It would take up too much time here to consider
each in detail,[69] but I would like to point out what
they reveal of the structure of initiation.

They use the stereotyped schema of "outside" and
"inside" to present the journey of the candidates. The
initial preaching was generally done in the streets or
some other public area. But catechesis was done in a
house since it was addressed only to those whose
conversion could be verified. In the same way, admission to baptism was not granted before an examination of the faith and the life of the catechumen.

In short, we find here again the dual structure, each
phase terminating in an examination without which
the following threshold could not be crossed.

The Clementine Stories

By way of example, let us consider one of the narratives that are found in the "Clementine Homelies." This is another popular story of the third century and it strongly resembles the apocryphal Acts. It tells of the conversion of a certain Clement.

One day in Alexandria, Clement was profoundly moved by the public preaching of Barnabas. Some Christians were proclaiming the Good News of Christ on the street corners to all who would listen as did the philosophers. As in Paul's time, their speeches aroused various reactions, most of which were hostile. Touched by grace, Clement tried to calm the threatening crowd and even to convince them. Then, to protect the preacher, he invited him home with him and profited from the occasion by having himself be instructed in the "first elements" of the truth.

The second scene of the story takes place in Caesarea in Palestine. The preacher introduces the new convert to Peter, the leader of the community, and witnesses to the sincerity of his faith and thus his capacity to receive catechesis. Clement continues:

> I asked for directions to Peter's house. When I was told, I presented myself at his door. The people of the house, having inspected me, wondered who I was and from whence I came. Then Barnabas came forward and, as soon as he saw me, flung his arms around my neck and shed many tears of joy. Then, taking me by the hand, he introduced me to Peter saying: "This is Peter whom I told you was the man best versed in the wisdom of God and whom I have never ceased telling about you. Go right in for I have told him in

all sincerity of the good that is in you, and I have also told him of your plan in such a way that he, too, wants very much to see you. You are a great present that I am bringing to him." With these words, he presented me saying, "Peter, this is Clement."

At my name, the excellent Peter came to me and kissed me. Then, having me sit down, he said immediately: "You did a beautiful and noble thing when, to honor the true God, without shame, without fear of the anger of the vulgar mob, you gave hospitality to Barnabas, the herald of truth. You shall be blessed. For, as you have welcomed as a host and loaded honors upon the ambassador of the truth, in its turn, the truth shall make you, who are a stranger, a citizen of its own city. It shall then be for you a great joy to see that, for a slight gesture of good will that you offer now—I mean the preference you give to the teaching—you shall be heir to inestimable eternal benefits. Do not bother to tell me of your disposition, since the truthful Barnabas has informed us of everything that concerns you, telling us almost every day something good about you. And, in a word, as to a true friend, if nothing prevents you, come with us on our journeys to share in the teaching of the truth that I shall distribute from city to city even to Rome itself.[70]

It is thus only after having manifested the sincerity of his conversion and with the guarantee of the one who evangelized him that Clement was admitted to the catechesis proper.

What is to be drawn from this story, which curiously recalls the conversion of Cornelius (Acts 10,11), is the very clear distinction that was made from then on between the period of evangelization and that of systematic instruction. The first period had to lead to faith.[71] The candidate was not admitted to the second period unless the Church had recognized the quality of his conversion, manifested concretely, and, if possible, guaranteed by the one who had been the instrument of that conversion.

We note here the same degree of seriousness regarding the examination that terminates the period of catechesis and allows the catechumen to be admitted to baptism. Thus, Clement was only baptized by Peter after having listened to his preaching for three months and having manifested his conversion of life.

The initiation ceremony was always preceded by a few days of fasting. The baptism took place at a pool in the presence of a few relatives and friends. Then everyone returned in procession to celebrate the eucharist with the brothers.[72]

Without wanting to force the probative value of each text, which would depend on their origins, an overall conviction emerges from these popular writings: in the third century, catechumenal practice had the same structure everywhere.

At the Dawn
of the Fourth Century

The Councils of 300-325

The information provided by some councils held in the beginning of the fourth century is less pictur-esque. But it is interesting to note that they confirm the catechumenal pedagogy described above. Even if they indicate a certain relaxation of discipline, they do show that the stage structure was still maintained and that the necessity of a certain period of formation was still affirmed.

Around 300 in Spain, the Council of Elvira witnesses to the maintenance of the requirements concerning the professions from which one had to refrain to be "received" into catechesis: prostitution (§44), carriage driving, and acting (§62). It shows that there was a rite of entrance into the catechumenate, the imposition of hands, by which one became a "Christian" (§39). It required two years of formation except for cases of urgency arising from illness (§42). While this is a little less than the prescriptions of Clement of Alexandria and Hippolytus, grave faults could prolong the cate-chumenal period up to three (§4) or five (§73) years or even to the moment of death (§68).

In 325, the Council of Nicea observed with regret that people were being baptized who had just passed from the pagan life to the faith and who had been only briefly instructed. Thus it laid down this prescription: "It is proper that in the future, this no longer be done since time is necessary for the catechumen (in view of baptism)"(§2).[73]

The Basilica at Tyre

At the end of this survey of the second and third centuries that has taken us from the birth through the expansion of the catechumenal discipline, an image suggests itself that well illustrates the situation we have arrived at. This is the image of the famous basilica built by Paulinus at Tyre after the peace of the Church. Eusebius praised it around 317.[74]

In a long description, the details of which are sometimes difficult to understand, Eusebius presents the different parts of this magnificent temple as the stages of Christian spiritual life. The various moments of the catechumenal journey emerge quite clearly.

The orator speaks first of the great vestibule of the East side that "invites, as it were, those who are strangers to the faith to turn their gaze to the first entrances" (§38). These are the responsibility of the guardians who are charged with "guiding those who enter" (§63).

Between the entrances and the temple itself, there is a large space surrounded by four porticos (§39). "It is there that have been placed the symbols of the sacred purifications," i.e. the fountains. This emplacement matches the requirements of "those who still need the first initiations" (§40) and who "are being advanced to the first approach to the letter of the four Gospels" (§63). This is an allusion to those who were formerly strangers to the faith but who have been converted and admitted to the group of catechumens.

Then, numerous vestibules are perceived that open to the entrances to the temple (§41). There are those who are "brought near to each side of the basilica: they are still catechumens and established in growth and progress but nevertheless are not far removed from the sight of the interior objects that the faithful contemplate" (§63). Probably these are the group of the "chosen ones" for the next baptism.

Finally, there are, at each side of the temple, "the places necessary for those who still have need of purification and ablutions conferred by water and the Holy Spirit (§45). There are initiated the "pure souls who are purified like gold by a divine bath" (§64).

Thus, from Justin to Eusebius, the evolution proceeded normally. That which was incipient in the New Testament developed progressively. The baptismal period, with its admission examination, was the first to be structured; then the catechumenal period itself was institutionalized and the entrance criteria were clearly formulated. The necessity of a preliminary evangelization period was emphasized.

The history of the catechumenate speaks for itself. In the four corners of the Mediterranean world, the Church introduced the requirement of a serious baptismal preparation. In the third century, we can see the most authentic form of the catechumenate: the witness of the martyrs, dialogue with Christians, and the life of the community awakened the faith of converts. The community then took charge of them and led them on the catechumenal journey. It took them in, instructed and formed them so that, by successive stages, they could enter into this new life that had to grow without ceasing and bear fruit. Would official recognition of the Church by the State sap this vitality?

72
Notes

[1] For this entire chapter, cf. Dujarier, *Parrainage des adultes,* pp. 173-344.

[2] Tertullian frequently uses the expression "seal of the faith" with variants: immersion is the sign of the faith *(obsignatio fidei) De paenitentia* VI, 16, CCL I, 331; *De idol.* 10,6,12; *Ad. Nat.* 8,16; baptism is also *signatio fidei, De pect.* 4,1; 24,2,3, CCL I, 231, p. 248. Tertullian speaks of the faith received and sealed at baptism *(suscepta atque signata), De corona* 11,4, CCL II, 1057. Very concisely, he says that water seals the faith *(fidem aqua signat), De praesc.* 36,5, CCL I, 217. In the same sense is the expression *obsignatio baptismi* by which the faith is lived, *De bapt.* 13,2, CCL I, 289; cf. *Adv. Marc.* I,28, *De anima,* I; see L. Villette, *Foi et sacrement,* Travaux de l'Institut catholique, vol. I, *Du Nouveau Testament à St. Augustin,* Paris, 1959, pp. 111-2. On baptism as seal of faith in the New Testament, cf. I. de la Potterie, *Biblica* 40, 1959, pp. 12-21: the affirmation that anointing does not allude to any rite of Christian origin is qualified.

[3] Tertullian, *De paenitentia* VI, 1-22; TD, edited by P. de Labriolle.

[4] Tertullian, *De bapt.* 18,1; SC 35, p. 91. It is necessary to study the use the Fathers of the Church made of these texts in arguing for the necessity of administering the sacraments with discernment. Cf. *Biblia Patristica,* which is in the process of being published by CNRS, Paris.

[5] Origen, *Hom. in Lev.* 6,2; GCS 6,361.

[6] Origen, *Hom. in Luc* 21,4; GCS 9,140; SC 87, pp. 294-5. Notes 2 and 3 in SC are very interesting with regard to the conversions in Origen. Origen specifies further on: "John speaks to the multitudes who came out to be baptized (Lk 3:7). If anyone wants to be baptized he must come out. To the extent that he remains in his first state, without changing his conduct and habits, he totally lacks the dispositions required to approach baptism. To understand what is meant by coming out to be baptized, it is necessary to consider the witness borne by the words of God to Abraham: Go from the country, etc. (Gen 12:1)"; *(Hom.* 22,5; see also 22,6). For Origen, the first stage consists of the departure from sin, from former habits, and from oneself. Cf. *Hom. in Jesu Nave* 4,1, SC 71, ed. A. Jaubert, pp. 148-9 and *Hom. in Num.* 26,4, SC 29, p. 501.

[7] Origen, *Hom. in Ezech.* 6,5; GCS 8,383.

[8] B. Capelle, "L'introduction du catéchuménat à Rome," *Recherches de théologie ancienne et médiévale* 5 (1933), pp. 129-54; J. Lebreton, "Le développement des institutions ecclésiastiques à la fin du second

siècle et au début du troisième," *Rech. sc. rel.* 24 (1934), pp. 129-64.

[9]"The Doctrine of the Twelve Apostles (Didache)": SC 248, VII,1: "after having said beforehand all that preceded, baptize. . . ." W. Rordof (p. 170, n. 3) does not accept the interpretation of Audet that this expression is a later interpolation.

[10]Hermas, "The Shepherd," SC 53(2), vis. III, 2,9 and 7,3.

[11]Justin, *The Writings of Justin Martyr and Athagoras,* translation by Maraes Dods, George Reith, and B. P. Pratten, Edinburgh, 1867, *Ante-Nicene Christian Library,* II. "The First Apology," 61-6; LC 3 or TD 1.

[12]Justin, "The Second Apology," 2; TD 1, p. 151.

[13]Justin, "The First Apology," 60; TD 1, p. 124.

[14]This was the case for Justin himself. Arrested and brought before the court, he said to the judge: "I stayed above a certain Martin, near the bath of Timothy. . . . I know of no other meeting place. To all those who wanted to find me there, I communicated the doctrine of truth," Act. Justin. III,3.

[15]Justin, "First Apology," 66,1.

[16]Ibid., 61,6-9.

[17]Ibid., 61,2.

[18]Ibid.

[19]Ibid., 66,1.

[20]"Didache," VII,4. *The Fathers of the Church,* vol. I, The Catholic University of America Press, Washington, D.C., 1947.

[21]Justin, "First Apology," 61,2.

[22]Ibid, 65-6.

[23]Cf. A. Mehat, *Etude sur les "Stromates" de Clément d'Alexandrie,* Seuil, Paris, 1966, pp. 62-70.

[24]I Strom. 19,4.

[25]VI Strom. 89,1-2.

[26]Ped. I,30,2.

[27]Ped. I,36,2-3.

[28]II Strom. 26,4-5.

[29]Mehat, p. 221. Contrary to Camelot, Mehat considers this text as a "certain allusion to the catechumenate." For inscription, see Mehat, p. 68.

[30]II Strom. 95,3-96,2.

[31]Mehat, p. 69. For what could be the baptismal rites of this period, see F. Sagnard, *Clément d'Alexandrie, Extraits de Théodote,* SC, 23, pp. 229-39: "Le baptême au deuxième siècle et son interprétation valentinienne."

[32]"Passion of SS. Perpetua and Felicity," I,1.

[33]Tertullian: *De praesc.* 41, 2 and 4. The first portion of this citation is the translation of T. Herbert Bindley, *Tertullian on the Testimony of the*

Soul and on the " Prescription of Heretics," SPCK, London, 1914, XLI, 2 and 4. We see here a clear indication of the three categories: the pagans, who did not enter; the catechumens, who listened; the faithful, who prayed.

[34]6,1.

[35]6,14. *Les classes* are the age groups subject to conscription.

[36]*Instructions,* II,5. Cf. the two studies by J. Durel, *Les Instructions de Commodien: Traduction et commentaire* and *Commodien: Recherches sur la doctrine, la langue et le vocabulaire du poète,* Leroux, Paris, 1912. CCL 128,43. We are preparing a study on the catechumenal usage of the word "tiro" and also on that of "proselyte of Christ." Significant instances can be found in Minucius Felix, Augustine, Quodvultdeus, Jerome, and Isidore of Seville.

[37]Cf. Dujarier, *Parrainage des adultes,* pp. 220-30, and Tertullian, *De paenitentia* VI, 1-22.

[38]Cf. Dujarier, *Parrainage des adultes,* pp. 231-2.

[39]*De bapt.* 20, 1 and 5.

[40]Ibid., 19, 1-2.

[41]On this subject, see the basic study of E. Dekkers, *Tertullianus en de Geschiedenis der Liturgie,* Bruges, 1947, pp. 163-216. Cyprian adds little that is new to what Tertullian writes about the history of the catechumenate, except for proof of the clericalization of catechists. On this subject, see Victor Saxer, *Vie liturgique et quotidienne à Carthage vers le milieu du IIIe siècle,* Vatican City, 1969, pp. 106-44.

[42]Tertullian, "The Chaplet," III, 2-3 *Tertullian: Disciplinary, Moral and Ascetical Works,* trans. by Rudolph Arbesmann et al., *The Fathers of the Church* XL, pp. 225-67.

[43]Hippolytus, *The Treatise on the Apostolic Tradition of St. Hippolytus of Rome,* ed. by Gregory Dix, SPCK, London 1968, p. 23.

[44]Ibid., pp. 24-28.

[45]Ibid., pp. 29-30.

[46]This way of doing things is confirmed by Origen. Cf. P. Nautin, *Origène: Homélies sur Jérémie. Tome 1,* SC 232, pp. 100-12.

[47]In the same way, the catechumens did not participate completely in the agape meal. They were present, but received only the bread of exorcism (§§27-28).

[48]Cf. Sagnard, *Clément d'Alexandrie,* p. 234.

[49]Hippolytus, p. 31.

[50]Cf. Dujarier, *Parrainage des adultes,* pp. 231-2.

[51]Hippolytus, 20, pp. 31-2.

[52]The description of the baptism and the eucharist that followed immediately is in §21. In Rome, as in Carthage, the neophytes were given milk and honey.

[53]Hippolytus, 23,12, p. 42. Note here the role the entire community has to play by its example in catechumenal education, chap. 41.

[54]Origen, *Hom. in Jer.* 4 ,3; GCS 3, ed. by E. Klostermann, p. 25; PG 13, (2) 880.

[55]Origen, *Hom. in Jesu Nave* 4,1; SC 71, ed. by A. Jaubert, pp. 148-9.

[56]Origen, *Hom. in Num.* 26,4; SC 29, p. 501. This biblical interpretation continued to the 4th century.

[57]Origen, *Contra Celsum,* 3,9, trans. by Henry Chadwick, Cambridge University Press, Cambridge, 1953, p. 133.

[58]Ibid., 3,55; pp. 165-6.

[59]Ibid., 3,15; p. 137.

[60]Ibid., 3,57-9; pp. 166-8.

[61]Ibid., 3,51; p. 163. In his work, "Against the Christians," Porphyry, a neo-Platonist contemporary of Origen, also witnesses to the existence of the catechumenate. With regard to the saying of Christ, " Feed my lambs, feed my sheep," he writes: "I suppose that the sheep are the faithful who have already advanced to the mystery of perfection, while the lambs mean the group of those who are still catechumens and who are nourished on the gentle milk of the doctrine" (Fragment 26).

[62]Origen, *Exhort. ad mart.,* 17, GCS 1,16; PG 11,585; *Exhortation to Martyrdom in Alexandrian Christianity,* trans. John Oulton and Henry Chadwick. Library of Christian Classics II, SCM, London, 1954.
The expression ἐνταῖς περὶ θεοσεβειάς συνθήκαις, which is here translated by "the agreements concerning religion" [Dujarier translates it in French by "les accords concernant votre attitude envers Dieu"], is significant: Συνθήκη has the sense of treaty, pact, alliance, accord in the strong sense, which has been established with God in the presence of the catechist; this word probably refers to the Shechem covenant, but it is not the term used by the LXX and the New Testament. Διαθήκη is the more common term of the same family.

[63]*Contra Celsum,* 3,51; p. 163.

[64]Ibid., 3,59; p. 168.

[65]Ibid.

[66]This parallelism between the stages of the catechumenate and those of the penitential system must be studied more thoroughly. For the 2nd century, traces are found in Hermas, Tertullian, and Cyprian, cf. A. d'Ales, *L'édit de Calliste,* pp. 54ff. and pp. 409-21. For the 3rd century, see the *Canonical Epistles* of Gregory Thaumaturgus, Migne Greek X, 1019-48.

[67]*Didascalia* 2,56. *The Didascalia Apostolorum in Syriac* by Margaret Dunlop Gibson, C. J. Clay and Sons, London, 1903,

[68]Ibid., 2,39,4-6; p. 55.

[69]Cf. Dujarier, *Parrainage des adultes,* pp. 297-312.

[70]*Hom. Clem.* 1,15-17; A. Siouville, *Les Homélies clémentines,* Paris, 1933.

[71] This journey to the faith could be very long, as can be seen in *Hom. Clem.* 15,10-11.

[72] Cf. Dujarier, *Parrainage des adultes,* pp. 312-28.

[73] Cf. Karl Josef von Hefele, *Histoire des conciles d'après les documents originaux,* trans. by Odon Delarc and Isidore Goschler, Paris. Latouzey, 1907-1952.

[74] *Histoire ecclésiastique,* X,IV, especially 37-65; SC 55.

*The Vicissitudes of the
Catechumenate
(Fourth-Sixth Centuries)*

THE Peace of Constantine, inaugurated in 313, marks an important turning point in the history of the Church. From an illegal religion, Christianity became legally tolerated, and this position was soon transformed into one of privileged liberty. The Christians rejoiced, and rightly so, in being able to profess their faith without being harassed. But this change brought with it grave new pastoral problems, especially when it became the official religion instead of being only a permitted religion.

I shall first take up these new problems, and we shall see that they were very far from indicating any qualitative progress. In the face of the laxity brought about by the facility created by the inception of a Christian regime, the bishops struggled to maintain the same authenticity in the administration of the sacraments that was known in the preceding missionary centuries.

The New Problems

IN a certain way, Origen regretted the passing of persecution, as we have seen, since the dangers abroad then compelled the catechumens to acquire faith of a very high quality. With the ease of the Constantinian era, quality unfortunately gave way to quantity. The decline of fervor manifested itself in defective motivation for conversion and in lengthy delays of baptism.

The Defective Motivation for Conversion

Defective motivation for conversion constitutes the most typical and most grave deviation of this period. When the obstacles confronting the baptismal candidates began to disappear, it became easier to enter the Church. The motivation for the step the new Christians were taking was far from always supernatural and often was grounded in self-interest.[1]

For example, sometimes the request for entry into the catechumenate was motivated by the desire to marry a Christian. Though this could well constitute a point of departure, it often led some to simulate a faith they did not have. These cases were not rare. Thus in Jerusalem, Cyril wanted to discriminate between the candidates who presented their names for baptism:

> Let there be no Simon among you, let there be no hypocrisy, let there be no idle curiosity to see what happens.
>
> Perhaps you had a different reason for

coming. For it is quite what might happen,
that a man should be wanting to advance his
suit with a Christian woman, and to that end
has come here. And there is the like possibili-
ty the other way round. Or often it may be a
slave that wanted to please his master.[2]

Cyril mentions the desire to please a master or a
friend, and some of these friends were in "high
places," so baptism was being requested for reasons
of political ambition. In fact, one became a "Christian" by virtue of the rite of entry into the catechumenate and this simple title facilitated access to public
positions. Ambrose, Bishop of Milan, courageously
denounced this practice:

And here is one who comes to the Church
because he is looking for honors under the
Christian emperors; he pretends to request
baptism with a simulated respect; he bows,
he prostrates; but he does not bend his
knees in spirit.[3]

What is serious in all this, says Ambrose, is hypocrisy
and duplicity:

To have a spouse who is refused them by
Christian parents—because they are pagans—
some simulate having the faith for a time,
then they show that they have confessed
exteriorly what they deny in their hearts.[4]

To these hypocrites, Augustine opposes the case of
someone who wants sincerely to become a Christian
and not "to obtain the hand of a Christian girl he
wants to marry."[5] This is why he advises constant
vigilance regarding the motives that lead someone to
request instruction:

For if he wishes to become a Christian in the hope of deriving some benefit from men whom he thinks he could not otherwise please, or to escape some injury at the hands of men whose displeasure or enmity he dreads, he in reality does not wish to become a Christian so much as he wishes to feign being one. . . . It is well, certainly to be informed, if possible, beforehand by those who know him of his state of mind and of the causes that have induced him to come and embrace religion. . . . If he has come with a counterfeit motive, desirous only of temporal advantages, or thinking to escape some loss, he will, of course, lie.[6]

The Postponement of Baptism

The deterioration of the motives for conversion increased the number of those asking to become Christians by entry into the catechumenate. At the same time, it triggered a second and inverse deviation: the indefinite postponement of baptism. What the "candidates" sought to obtain was simply the title of "Christian"; they had no true desire for baptism.

This problem also arose for children whose Christian parents entered them into the catechumenate but who were never given any further instruction in the Christian faith. Therefore, they remained catechumens for life unless they underwent a true conversion when they were older. Basil, Gregory of Nazianzus, Augustine, and many others were in this category. Augustine, when he was very young, had been "signed with the sign of the cross of (Christ) and seasoned with his salt." During an illness, baptism was discussed, but when his health improved he again delayed the reception of the sacrament. He finally was baptized at the age of thirty-three, that is, after his conversion.[7]

What should we think of these adults who became Christians without any desire to request baptism? Though they bore the name, they were not in fact Christians since they were not converted.

The bishops did not cease protesting vigorously against such abuses. In the West, it was customary on Epiphany for preachers to try to awaken these slumbering catechumens so that they would "give their names" at the beginning of Lent with a view to baptism on the coming Easter. But their appeals often remained fruitless. The sadness of a bishop like Ambrose was great when, in commenting on the miraculous catch of Lk 4:5, he noted that none had responded:

> I, too, Lord, I know that for me it is dark when you do not command. No one has yet inscribed, it is still night for me. I put out the net of the word at Epiphany, and I have not yet taken anything.[8]

Basil earnestly invited those already "conceived" (by entrance into the catechumenate) to accept the sacrament that would "bring them into the world":

> Catechized since you were young, do you still not give your accord to the truth? You who do not cease studying, have you not yet arrived at knowledge? You who are tasting life, explorer until old age, will you finish by becoming Christian? . . . Better not to end by being surprised while making promises longer than your life. You do not know what

tomorrow will bring, do not promise what is not yours. We are calling you to life, man; why do you flee from this call? . . . If I would distribute gold to the assembly, you would not say to me, "I shall come tomorrow and you will give to me tomorrow"; but you would claim your share of the distribution and you would take it ill if you were passed over; and when the great dispenser offers you, not shining matter, but purity of the soul, you make up excuses and enumerate motives, while you should come to the distribution. . . . Depend on the Lord. Give your name, inscribe in the Church. . . . Inscribe in this book, in order to participate in the inscription in that of heaven. Instruct yourself, study the evangelical constitution. . . . Put sin to death; be crucified with Christ; carry all your love to the Lord.[9]

Gregory of Nazianzus worked unceasingly to prove that there was absolutely no valid reason to defer baptism:

Let us be baptized today so as not to be forced to do it tomorrow. Let us not delay the blessing, as though it would cause us harm. Let us not wait to sin more so that we might be forgiven more. This would be to involve Christ in an unworthy commercial speculation: to burden ourselves with more than we can carry, to run the risk of seeing his ship totally perish and to lose in a shipwreck all the fruit of grace we did not know how to consume.[10]

Gregory of Nyssa also denounced as detestable the

motives alleged: under a false show of humility, it was actually a refusal to renounce sin that held back these people who were comparable to the unprofitable servant who hid his talent.[11] "It is not sufficient to be conceived," wrote Augustine, "it is necessary to be born again to come to eternal life."[12]

With the same vigor, John Chrysostom fought against the custom of postponing baptism until one was *in extremis:*

> Is it not the utmost stupidity to postpone the gift? Listen you catechumens and you who put off your own salvation until the last gasp![13]

Such inertia, moreover, constituted a scandal that was highly amusing to the pagans. If one truly believed in the greatness of the sacrament, why wait until one was ill? This would be like a soldier who waits for the war to be over before going to battle.[14]

In reality, this custom reveals the depths to which the catechumenate had fallen. The title of catechumen had lost its profound significance, since it no longer corresponded to a true conversion, so the catechumenate itself declined. Scandalized by this massive indifference, the bishops hurried the catechumens into baptism, with all the attendant dangers of formalism. Much was said about catechumens in this period, but though there were many catechumens, there were few true converts. Whether it was a question of children who had not yet given their assent to the truth even though they had been instructed in the rudiments of the faith, or adults who entered the Church for defective motives, the title no longer corresponded to the reality it expressed formerly. Nevertheless, pastors never forgot the theological exigencies of an authentic sacramental ministry.

The Permanent Concern for Authenticity

IT is instructive to consider the efforts of the Fathers of the fourth and fifth centuries to prevent a fatal decline. They were the first to recognize a certain weakening not only in the delay of baptism by adults but also in the temptation of priests to admit to baptism those who pretended to have the faith and who did not live in a Christian way. Faced with this abuse, they did not hesitate to call upon the traditional doctrine according to which salvation is only granted in the sacrament to those having the faith and living in conformity to that faith. From this double requirement followed the necessity of a catechumenal discipline.

The Necessity of Real Faith

The bishops first stressed that faith is intimately bound to the sacrament[15]: no sacrament may be administered if it is absent.

> Faith and Baptism are two modes of salvation, of kindred origin and inseparable. For on the one hand faith is perfected through baptism, and on the other hand baptism is founded on faith.[16]

So wrote Basil of Caesarea. This theme recurred often in his preaching:

> Go, said the Lord, teach all nations, baptize them in the name of the Father, the Son, and the Spirit. Baptism is, in fact, the seal of the

86

faith, and the faith is a bond with the Divinity.
Therefore, it is necessary first to believe, and
then to be signed by baptism.[17]

Referring likewise to the command of Jesus Christ
before his ascension, Athanasius and Jerome stressed
the same requirement:

The Savior commanded not only to baptize,
he said first "to teach" and then "to baptize,"
so that teaching may give birth to the proper
faith and that, with the faith, we may be
initiated by the sacrament.[18]

The Apostles first taught all the nations:
once they taught them, they gave them ablu-
tion with water. Indeed, the body cannot
receive the sacrament of baptism if the soul,
before all else, has not welcomed the truth of
the faith.[19]

One of the objectives of the catechumenate is to
increase the faith of those in whom "the grace of the
faith is not yet sufficient to obtain the Kingdom of
God."[20]

Of itself, this requirement of a certain maturity in
the faith to receive baptism suffices to justify serious
prebaptismal catechesis. But there is another requirement that confirms the utility of a period of preliminary formation: the faith that gives access to the font
of new birth is not a dead faith, it is a living faith
animated by an efficacious love.

The Necessity of a Life That Conforms
to the Faith

Augustine wrote an entire treatise, "On Faith and
Works," to denounce the practice of baptizing sinners

that was developing in some places:

> There are certain persons who are of the opinion that everybody without exception must be admitted to the font of rebirth which is in Christ Jesus our Lord, even those who, notorious for their crimes and flagrant vices, are unwilling to change their evil and shameful ways, and declare frankly (and publicly) that they intend to continue in their state of sin.[21]

And it is not sufficient to say: "Then he will be taught how evil it is and, after baptism, he will be instructed to reform his morals," since such is contrary to the practice of the Church:

> With the help of our Lord God, let us diligently beware henceforth of giving men a false confidence by telling them that if only they will have been baptized in Christ, no matter how they will live in the faith, they will arrive at eternal salvation.[22]

This is the same fundamental theme that recurs in many of the Lenten sermons of this period. Baptismal life can permeate only those who have rejected all hypocrisy and who already are accustomed to live in conformity with the Gospel. The following is from Cyril of Jerusalem:

> For though you be present here in the body, that is no use if your heart be not here as well. Once upon a time there came to the font Simon the Sorcerer. He was baptized, but he was not enlightened, for while his body went under the water, his heart let not in the light of the Spirit. He plunged his body

and came up, but in his soul, he was neither buried with Christ nor did he rise again with him. . . . But if you just continue in your evil disposition, I have cleared myself of telling you, but you cannot expect to receive God's grace. For though the water will receive you, the Holy Spirit will not.[23]

In his second baptismal instruction, John Chrysostom drew the practical conclusion from this traditional teaching:

I have said it before, I say it now, and I shall say it again and again: unless a man has corrected the defects of his character and has developed a facility for virtue, let him not be baptized. Consider your soul as a portrait that you have painted. Before the Holy Spirit comes to apply his divine brush, erase your bad habits.[24]

Gregory of Nyssa did not hesitate to affirm that baptism conferred on a poorly prepared candidate is not only inefficacious, it is also an insult to God himself:

If the washing is applied to the body, while the soul does not wash away the stains of its passions, but the life after initiation is of the same character as the initiate life, even though it be a bold thing to say, yet I will say it and not draw back, in such cases the water is water, and the gift of the Holy Spirit nowhere appears in what takes place: the turpitude of the soul dishonours the image of God.[25]

At the beginning of the sixth century, the same theme recurs in the Sermons of Cesarius of Arles to those to be baptized:

> It is a good thing you are seeking, a great thing, the highest bliss, eternal happiness. For this reason I admonish you with God's help devoutly to prepare both your bodies and your hearts, because what you are asking is very great. In truth if God wanted to offer you individual silk garments, you would not be able to accept them with filthy, dirty hands. How much more so, then, when He deigns to give His own self to you, should you not receive Him except in a heart that has been cleansed by faith? If, according to the Lord's precept "people do not pour new wine into old wineskins," how will any man be able to receive God Himself if he has been unwilling to cleanse himself entirely of his old way of life?[26]

Thus, from the fourth to the sixth century, the bishops firmly maintained the theological principles of the sacramental ministry, while the Peace of Constantine was threatening to make it too easy for the catechumens. How did the institution of the catechumenate adapt to the new situation? I turn now to this problem.

The description of the catechumenate around the year 400 shows how the Church tried to preserve the proper balance between mercifulness and laxity. Augustine clearly saw that Donatism, with its tendency to construct a "church of the pure," was as dangerous as the abandonment of ecclesiastical discipline. In pastoral practice, it is necessary to join firmness with goodness, without becoming "torpid in the name of patience nor violent under the pretext of zeal."[27]

The Catechumenate from 350 to 420

WHAT were the stages of the catechumenate in the years between 350 and 420? The following survey shows clearly that the catechumenate proper weakened and that a new structuring of Lent was implemented to remedy it.

The vocabulary then employed seems to indicate that the catechumenal structure was still vital. Some homilies show that conversion was conceived as a journey in four stages: first, when we were pagans, we were converted by the proclamation of the Gospel; then we became catechumens; then there was the intensive formation of the elect during Lent; then we were baptized. This is the obvious sense of what Gregory of Elvira writes about Noah's Ark:

> The Lord ordered Noah to make an ark with three rooms as a figure of the Church. First the word of the Law penetrates into the catechumen as through the entry of a body. Then the mystery of the sacrament enters into the *competens* to hide itself in the secret of his soul as in a linen shop. In the third place, in the faithful, the Holy Spirit arrives at the summit via the degrees of virtue as in the upper floors of a house.[28]

This is also expressed in the picturesque and very beautiful text of Augustine comparing the new Christian to wheat that is threshed, gathered, ground into flour, kneaded, and finally made into bread:

> You have been led to the threshing floor of
> the Lord, you have been ground by oxen, that
> is, by those who have announced the Gospel
> to you. Once catechumens, you were gar-
> nered. You have been given names, you have
> begun to be milled by fasts, by exorcisms.
> Afterwards, you came to the fountain, you
> have been baptized, you have become one
> single body. You have been baked by the fire
> of the Holy Spirit, and you have become the
> bread of the Lord.[29]

Thus the same stages are spoken of as in the third
century and always with the same vocabulary. But
what reality was behind this way of speaking?

Was There Still an Entry into the Catechumenate?

We recall how seriously admission to catechesis was
taken during the third century, the examination that
permitted the postulant to enter the Church after
having proved the quality of his approach. In the
fourth century, it seems that the rite still existed but
that it rarely represented the sanction of a profound
and sincere conversion.

It was customary for parents to present their children to the priest so they could become catechumens.
The essential rite was the signing,[30] which in Africa
was accompanied by the tasting of salt.[31] The practice
with adults, however, requires closer examination.

There are quite a number of documents that witness
to the existence of the rite itself—the sign of the cross
with an imposition of hands—but it seems they were
only interested in miraculous conversions.[32] The role

of the Church and of Christians seems to have been quite insignifcant.

Three works from the East indicate that the practice attested to by Hippolytus was still in force: these are the *Canons of Hippolytus* (Egypt, ca. 360), the *Testament of our Lord Jesus Christ* (Syria, fourth century), and the *Apostolic Constitutions* (Syria, fourth-fifth century), which speak of an entrance examination for the catechumenate. But these three documents were directly based on the *Apostolic Tradition* of Hippolytus. They recall an ideal but do not witness to a practice except in the few details in which they differ from their source.[33]

There is only one document that can be considered a witness of value: *De catechizandis rudibus* of Augustine. He described the rite of entry into the catechumenate in these terms:

> After the instruction you should ask him whether he believes these things and desires to observe them. And when he answers that he does, you should of course sign him, with due ceremony, and deal with him in accordance with the custom of the Church.[34]

The administration of this rite supposes a preliminary profession of faith: the candidate had to signify his adherence to the presentation of the whole of the Christian message, which he had just heard, and to renounce the service of idols.[35]

Thus the principle was secure, but we must recognize that there was not always sufficient evangelization. If some had personally read the Scriptures,[36] many others came without any preparation, and sometimes even with defective motives.[37] How could a pre-catechesis that was reduced to a meeting that did not exceed two hours work an effective transformation?

The situation had certainly changed with respect to the preceding century. If, despite the great amount of patristic literature we have from the fourth century, we have so few witnesses to a serious admission examination for the catechumenate, it is because, from this time on, the rite was conferred too readily. It was used as a lure, while it should have sanctioned a conversion! And without a true conversion, it was an empty gesture. It is easy to see why such "catechumens" were so little concerned with forming themselves for baptism.

What Remained of the Catechumenate Itself?

The duration of catechesis varied a great deal. The catechumens with a slight degree of conviction postponed baptism indefinitely. Those who did decide to proceed were baptized rather quickly.

At the beginning of the fourth century in Spain,[38] as we have seen, the bishops still required two years. But around the year 400, it seems there was no specified minimum. Moreover, the catechumenate, properly speaking, no longer existed. The catechumens participated or not in the Liturgy of the Word according to the degree of their conviction. They were not closely supervised by the authorities in structured groups. The Church seemed to be more preoccupied with "pushing" spiritless candidates to baptism than with moderating, with a long period of testing, the zeal of the rare candidate who was in too much of a hurry. And if a candidate was particularly well disposed, he was accepted for initiation very quickly.[39]

Nevertheless, the Church continued to maintain in principle the necessity of a certain amount of time for the catechumenate, as Augustine states:

> What, moreover, is all that time for, during which they hold the name and place of catechumens, except to hear what the faith and pattern of Christian life should be, so that first they may prove themselves and then eat of the Bread of the Lord and drink of the Chalice . . . . This training actually goes on during all that time which the Church has beneficially appointed for the candidates for admission to the catechumenate. Their study, too, becomes far more earnest and intensive during the period in which they are called *competentes,* that is, when they have already given in their names for the reception of baptism.[40]

Thus the principle. But what was the reality? The catechumens who were unconvinced were not obliged to attend sermons often, if one can judge from the content of the sermons given at the beginning of Lent. And to those who had submitted their names for baptism, it was still necessary to preach conversion, purity of intention, and transformation of morals!

As the terms he used in his *Procatechesis* indicate, Cyril of Jerusalem addressed himself to candidates who probably never followed a serious catechumenate. Even if they had attended a few instructions, they certainly had yet to grasp the vital exigencies of the Word of God:

> For we, Christ's ministers, have received each one of you. If you think of us as, figuratively, his door-keepers, then we have left the door unfastened. There has been

96

> nothing to stop you coming here with your
> soul covered in the mire of sins, with purpose
> anything but pure. . . . Let us say that your
> soul is wrapped in avarice. When you come
> back, let it wear a different dress: I do not
> mean on top of the old one, but with the old
> one taken off. Strip off, I beg, fornication and
> uncleanness and put on that brilliant robe,
> self-discipline. . . . You have a long period of
> grace, forty days for repentance. . . . You
> were called catechumen, which means one
> into whom something is dinned from with-
> out. You heard of some hope, but you did
> not know what. You heard mysteries without
> understanding anything. You heard Scrip-
> tures without plumbing their depth. It is not
> dinned in, any more, but whispered.[41]

Only thirty days before the baptism, John Chrysostom was still obliged to invite the candidates to
thorough moral conversion. Would he have done this
if the prior catechumenate had been lived seriously?

> Young athletes, the stadium is open, there
> are the spectators on the tiers of the amphi-
> theatre, in front of them is the leader of the
> games. Then, there is no middle ground,
> either you fall like a coward and leave cov-
> ered with shame, or you act bravely and win
> the crown and the prize. In the same way,
> these thirty days are the time of struggle, of
> apprenticeship, of exercise.[42]

Indeed, this transformation of life is urgent! The
orator feels it and he is eager to see concrete results,
for, six days later, he says:

It has only been a few days, my brothers, since I have spoken to you and I come already to claim the fruits of my instructions. Indeed, we speak not only for your ears, but for your spirits, in order that they may retain our words and that you let (us) see it through your works, or rather not us, but God who knows the depths of your hearts. We also appeal to our catechetical instructions because it is necessary that even in our absence the echo of our words resounds in your souls. . . . You, therefore, who have received our words and have put them into practice, persevere and advance. And you who have not yet began the work, start from now on so that your efforts will keep you from being accused of negligence in the future.[43]

Such words cannot be found on the lips of Hippolytus or Origen a few weeks before baptism. In the fourth century, the catechumenate was not what it was a hundred years earlier. The catechumens do not seem to have been convinced. And even when they came to the Church, the preaching does not seem to have penetrated: their faith was no longer capable of transforming their lives. No special institutions supported them or placed demands on them.

It was precisely to remedy this grave lacuna of a lax catechumenate that the Church developed Lent as the time of baptismal formation.

Inscription at the Beginning of Lent

To safeguard the requirements for admission to baptism, the custom was established to have Lent be a time of intense formation. The so-called catechumens, if they agreed to submit their names, were to accomplish in a few weeks the vital transformation that, in the preceding century, required two or three years.

The Lenten period opened with the solemn inscription of the names. This was seen as a renewal of the ceremony of entrance into the catechumenate, a ceremony that had not been founded on true conversion. But, after the years of slumber, were the catechumens really ready to follow Christ?

The candidates who had finally decided to receive the sacrament enrolled for baptism on the coming Easter. This ceremony is described in detail by Egeria, who gives the practice of the Jerusalem Church of around the year 400:

> I feel I should add something about the way they instruct those who are to be baptized at Easter. Names must be given in before the first day of Lent, which means that a presbyter takes down all the names before the start of the eight weeks for which Lent lasts here, as I have told you. Once the priest has all the names, on the second day of Lent at the start of the eight weeks, the bishop's chair is placed in the middle of the Great Church, the Martyrium, the presbyters sit in chairs on either side of him, and all the clergy stand. Then one by one those seeking baptism are brought up, men coming with their fathers and women with their mothers. As they come in one by one, the bishop asks their neighbours questions about them: "Is this person leading a good life? Does he respect his parents? Is he a drunkard or a boaster?" He asks about all the serious human vices. And if

his inquiries show him that someone has not committed any of these misdeeds, he himself puts down his name; but if someone is guilty he is told to go away, and the bishop tells him that he is to amend his ways before he may come to the font. He asks the men and the women the same questions. But it is not too easy for a visitor to come to baptism if he has no witnesses who are acquainted with him.[44]

According to this document, the examination of those who were henceforth called *competentes* apparently was carefully done. The life of the candidate was investigated. But, in these liturgies in front of all the people, did the rite truly match the requirements it signified? The same thing is found in the description Theodore of Mopsuestia gives of the ceremony as it was performed in Antioch at the same period:

Thus whoever desires to have access to the gift of holy baptism, let him present himself to the Church of God. He will be received by the one who is responsible for this, according to the custom that is established to inscribe those who want to be baptized. He shall inform himself of the morals. This function is performed for those who are baptized by the one who is called the guarantor. Now, he who is charged with the duty inscribes your name in the book of the Church and also adds that of the witness or of the pastor of the city or the parish.[45]

This text, which also gives us information on sponsorship, still requires some reserve. We have already seen that John Chrysostom received candidates only thirty days before baptism. Close examination of the homilies of Theodore of Mopsuestia yields support for the opinion that the ceremony of inscription did not take place on the first Sunday of Lent, but two weeks before Easter,[46] which confirms the observation made above. At the beginning of Lent, the candidates were just barely converted. Their liturgical inscription, which supposed a sincere and proven conversion, could not be done prematurely. Thus, one was obliged to postpone it more and more, at the risk of reducing the forty days, already too brief, to a few weeks or even a few days.[47]

Significant here is the question that the *Canons of Hippolytus* (ca. 360) put on the lips of the bishop. It would never have been asked on the eve of baptism in the third century:

> Are you hesitant, or held back for a reason or for fear of what people might say? For no one makes light of the kingdom of heaven, but it is given to those who love it with all their heart.[48]

The Lenten Retreat

Lent was a time of doctrinal and moral formation. Regular attendance at the sermons had to correspond to moral conversion. Continuous and thorough catechetical instruction was provided for the candidates. Egeria gives us a beautiful description of what was done in the Jerusalem Church:

> They have here the custom that those who are preparing for baptism during the season of the Lenten fast go to be exorcized by the clergy first thing in the morning, directly after

the morning dismissal in the Anastasis. As soon as that has taken place, the bishop's chair is placed in the Great Church, the Martyrium, and all those to be baptized, the men and the women, sit round him in a circle. There is a place where the fathers and mothers stand, and any of the people who want to listen (the faithful, of course) can come in and sit down, though not the cate- chumens, who do not come in while the bishop is teaching.

His subject is God's Law; during the forty days he goes through the whole Bible, begin- ning with Genesis, and first relating the literal meaning of each passage, then interpreting its spiritual meaning. He also teaches them at this time all about the resurrection and the faith. And this is called *catechesis*. After five weeks' teaching they receive the Creed, whose content he explains article by article in the same way as he explained the Scriptures, first literally and then spiritually. Thus all the people in these parts are able to follow the Scriptures when they are read in church, since there has been teaching on all the Scriptures from six to nine in the morning all through Lent, three hours' catechesis a day. . . . So the dismissal is at nine, which makes three hours' teaching a day for seven weeks.[49]

To these catechetical lessons on Scripture and the Creed,[50] some Churches also added catechesis on the Our Father.[51] Toward the end of Lent, the two ceremonies called the "traditions," of giving the Creed and the Our Father to the baptismal candidates, took place. In Jerusalem, the submission of the candidates to the Creed was customarily done on Palm Sunday.[52] During this formation, God strengthens those to be baptized with sacramentals and particularly the daily exorcisms of which Egeria speaks.

All the liturgical rites and penitential signs performed during Lent, explained Quodvultdeus, an African bishop, are to be considered as nutrition given by Mother Church to the children she carries in her womb and whom she will bring forth on Easter:

> All the sacramental rites done for you by the ministry of the servants of God, the exorcisms, the prayers, the psalms, the insufflations, the hair-shirt, the bowings of the head, the genuflections . . . all this, I have said, is the nourishment that your mother gives you in her womb so that she can bring you to rebirth in the water of baptism and present you to Christ exulting with joy.[53]

In addition to the daily exorcisms administered by the clerics to the *competentes,* there was the final solemn exorcism, including an anointing that was done by the bishop. By this rite, God scrutinizes the candidates' hearts to eliminate the very last impurity. But the God who expels the evil spirit only works in hearts that have decided to live according to the Gospel. This is why Augustine insisted on the personal participation necessary for this ceremony, which is a true combat.[54]

Theodore of Mopsuestia describes this ceremony with an extended commentary on the symbolism of the customs (from nudity to the linen veil) and the positions (standing, hands outstretched toward God, kneeling). It is the definitive renunciation of Satan who held us in bondage; it is a contract binding us to Christ, the sole master of life.

> After having said: "I renounce Satan, his angels, his service, his vanity and all his worldly errors," you say: "and I bind myself by vow; I believe and am baptized in the name of the Father, and of the Son and of the Holy Spirit." The same when you say: "I renounce" and that you abstain absolutely, you show that henceforth you will never turn back, that henceforth you will no longer take pleasure in his company; so, too, when you say: "I bind myself by vow," you show that you will remain resolutely near to God and that you from then on will be steadfastly with him, that in no way any longer will you turn from him and that you will consider it henceforth more precious for you than all things to live and converse with him and to conform to his laws. . . .
>
> This consignation with which you are now signed is the sign that you have been marked henceforth as a lamb of God, as a soldier of the King of heaven. . . .
>
> First, of course, you are naked, since this is how captives and slaves are; but when you have been marked, you place a linen veil on your head, which is the sign of the free state to which you have been called.[55]

The Baptism

Already begun, the celebration of baptism entered into its essential phase in Holy Week.

The baptismal ceremony as such began on the day before Easter and unfolded throughout the Vigil. The feast of the resurrection of Christ is indeed the most appropriate time for the celebration of the sacrament by which we die and rise again with Jesus.[56]

It is not my purpose here to describe the rites in detail.[57] I only want to stress that this feast of initiation, which consisted of the three sacraments of baptism, confirmation, and the eucharist in one whole, was a feast of the entire Christian community. Here is how John Chrysostom described the joy of this Paschal celebration:

> When the neophytes emerge from the sacred waters, all the congregation embraces them, greets them, gives them the kiss, congratulates them, and shares their joy at, having once been slaves and captives, becoming in an instant free men, sons invited to the royal table. As soon as they ascend from the waters, they are led to the awesome table, the source of a thousand favors, they taste the body and the blood of the Lord and become the dwelling of the Spirit: they are clothed with Christ himself and, as such, everywhere they go, they appear, like terrestial angels, as radiant as a burst of sunlight.[58]
>
> The Church of God is joyful because of her children. Indeed, like a loving mother who, seeing her children around her, rejoices, exults, and no longer contains her joy, so too the Church, in her spiritual maternity, when she gazes on her own children, is joyful and delighted, seeing herself as a fertile field full of spiritual grain.[59]

From then on, the newly baptized were called "faithful" because their faith had been sealed by the Holy Spirit.[60] But it is not enough to preserve it, it must be developed ceaselessly:

> Therefore, imitate God according to your capacity and according to his command, in all he has confided to you. Add to the sanctity you have received; enhance and polish more the justice and grace of your baptism; act like Saint Paul who increased each day—through his labors, his activity, and his zeal—the riches that God communicated to him.[61]

A New Life

During the week that followed the celebration of baptism, the neophytes returned each day to the church to hear a commentary on the sacraments they had just received. This is the mystagogical catechesis, which, according to Egeria, aroused a great deal of enthusiasm:

> The newly-baptized come into the Anastasis, and any of the faithful who wish to hear the Mysteries; but, while the bishop is teaching, no catechumen comes in, and the doors are kept shut in case any try to enter. The bishop relates what has been done, and interprets it, and, as he does so, the applause is so loud that it can be heard outside the Church.[62]

What did the bishop talk about? In some churches, the preacher explained the various rites of initiation to help the newly baptized become aware of the reality they had experienced. In addition, this catechesis was directed more to the moral requirements of an authentic Christian life.[63] Indeed, the whole purpose of catechumenal education was to lead to a new birth. Thus, far from being the end of a journey, baptism is the beginning of a life with and in Christ:

> The Apostle says: "All you who have been baptized in Christ, you have put on Christ." Let the newly baptized from now on do everything and act everywhere as permanently dwelling in Christ, creator of the universe and master of our nature. And when I say Christ, I say also the Father and the Holy Spirit.[64]
>
> Imitate him, you also, I implore you, and you will be called neophytes not only for two, three, ten, or twenty days, but you will still merit this name after ten, twenty, or thirty years, and in fact for all of your lives.[65]

This is the meaning of the white garment with which the neophyte was clothed. It invited him to live his life in imitation of Christ, a life that will be a permanent witness to men:

> It is right that those who have Christ, not as represented by a garment but as permanently residing in their souls, and with Christ his Father and the presence of the Holy Spirit, give proof of a firm confidence and show everyone, by the correctness of their conduct and the probity of their lives, that they bear the royal image.[66]

Evaluation of the Fourth and Fifth Centuries

WHAT lessons can we draw from the evolution that is apparent from this brief survey of the catechumenal practice of the fourth and fifth centuries? A critical judgment must involve balancing both its positive and negative aspects.

The Negative Side

In relation to the practice of the third century, two things indicate a regression in the quality of the catechumenal ministry.

First, the catechumenate as such had disappeared. I have listed the causes, here are the consequences:

The entry into the catechumenate lost its character of being a step taken in faith. Since the evangelization had not been thorough enough, the candidates were not ready to "hear the word." They were not truly converted. They saw the Church they entered as a simple institution from which they expected only advantages. They were ignorant of the very principle of its existence, which is communion in faith and because of which only those who believed in Christ could be admitted. This deficiency of faith matched an indifference toward evangelical conversion. The fervor of the communities slackened and baptism was postponed indefinitely.

It is important to understand that the devaluation of the entry into the catechumenate is at the source of the devaluation of the catechumenate, for catechu-

menal formation cannot be experienced authentically
except by subjects who actually believe in Christ, who
have vitally grasped the demands of the call of the
Lord, and who have decided to proceed to baptism.
Faith of conversion implies desire for the sacrament.
Where it does not exist, everything is false and even
the best organization cannot compensate for it. John
Chrysostom thought that it was better to leave the
catechumenate than to bear hypocritically a title that
no longer corresponded to anything:

> Do you still doubt the divinity of Jesus
> Christ? Then leave, listen no more to the holy
> word and remove your name from the list of
> the catechumens. But if you believe in Christ,
> God and man, and if you are clear about
> religion, then why these delays, these post-
> ponements, and this negligence?[67]

Second, the true meaning of baptism became
blurred. While access to the sacrament was a matter of
"election" for Hippolytus, it seems that from this time
on some catechumens looked on it as a right. This is
far from the teaching of Tertullian. Certainly, the
bishops still reaffirmed the baptismal requirements,
but their efforts reflect precisely the false conception
many had of baptism. The principles were maintained,
but the practice was totally different.

Baptism was even considered by some as a kind of
insurance, which one took out at the very last moment
to get the maximum advantage for the minimum cost,
or as an arduous obligation one had to accept to avoid
hell. Gregory of Nazianzus condemned these notions:

> I know three ways of salvation: that of
> slaves, that of mercenaries, that of sons.
> Slave, fear blows; mercenary, look only to

109

profit. But raise yourself to the dignity of son, love your Father with respect. Do good because of the beauty of obedience, even gratuitously, to your father, while not forgetting that your reward is the pleasure of your father.[68]

The abuses emphasized by the Fathers arose from the very position of the Church in the world. Because of the liberty it enjoyed from 313 on and the privileges it acquired, it ran the danger of being contaminated by the mentality of the world and of forgetting that it had to be the "soul of the world" by living evangelically.[69] In spite of the tremendous efforts of some bishops, the evangelical life had become confined to monks alone. This should make us realize that the renewal of the catechumenate cannot be accomplished without a profound renewal of all of our Christian communities.

The Positive Side

It is to the credit of the pastors of this period that they organized the Lenten catechumenate with the intention of remedying the situation. The pagan world had provided the Church with a remarkable group of men trained in classical culture and as gifted for administration and speculation as for liturgical organization.

We have seen how the Lenten period was structured in function of direct preparation for baptism. In principle, the requirements for entrance into the catechumenate were presented eight weeks before Easter, and these long weeks were the framework for an intense and serious formation of those to be baptized. The attempt was thereby made to accomplish in a condensed form what was done during the normal stages of the former catechumenate.[70]

But the suppression of the "real" catechumenate for the Lenten catechumenate led to a fatal decline. The evolution was inevitable: when the liturgical signs no longer correspond to the human journey, when they are deprived of their normal support, when they no longer express a lived reality, then there is no longer the necessity of extending them in time. The very notion of a journey toward baptism was progressively weakened and the spread of the custom of infant baptism caused it to disappear completely, even though in the beginning the parents of the infants to be baptized were required to follow the catechumenal stages with the *competentes*.[71]

In other respects the mystique of the preceding centuries became more conscious in the effort to compensate for the laxity of the ministry. One image in particular was often used by the Fathers to explain the necessity of the catechumenal stages: the gestation of a child in the womb of its mother.[72] The signing at the entry into the catechumenate, which ratified the first act of faith, was seen as the conception of the convert in the womb of the Church. But who has just started to live is still not ready to come into the world by the birth of baptism, and it would be criminal to send forth a being who is still too frail to survive. This is why, during the catechumenate—the period of gestation—the Church, like a good mother, nourishes by teaching and liturgical rites the one who will be reborn in the baptismal font.

Nonetheless, it is well to stress that the notion of stages is fundamental to Christian initiation. Of vital necessity are not only a serious catechesis but also an efficacious probation period. And there must also be a stage preliminary to catechesis, a stage that permits the seed of faith to be offered to those capable of welcoming it in their hearts and their lives.

The stages of the sacrament must coincide with those of the faith. In no case may the sacramental rites be performed without a true education in the faith. And, inversely, maturation in the faith has to be able to profit from the riches that Christ has provided in his liturgy.

While we may well rejoice in the modern restoration of the ritual of baptism by stages, let us beware of improperly sacramentalizing it.

Conclusion

I have given a great deal of attention to the most vital period of the catechumenate, the third century, at the risk of passing too cursorily over the period when the liturgical stages were solidified into ritual and progressively lost their function. This process of solidification, which began in the fourth century, merits a study of its own. Such a study could explain the process of the codification of the laws regarding sponsorship, which occurred because vital and spontaneous sponsorship was disappearing. A remedy was sought by establishing guarantors to support and encourage the catechumen. The institution of a solid structure gave the illusion of having revivified it. But, divorced from life, evolution froze and the structure remained until the day when, devitalized, it collapsed of its own accord.

Let us try now to determine the significance of the catechumenal experience of the first six centuries of the history of the Church.

Conversion and Faith

The sacramental act has nothing magical or automatic about it. Certainly, there is a totally gratuitous supernatural gift from God. But the Church, which has been charged with communicating this gift, cannot transmit it indiscriminately,[73] for an active disposition is required of the person who welcomes it.

To respect this principle as far as baptism is concerned, the Church has always demanded an authentic and living faith from the candidate. It has agreed to confer the sacrament without prior verification of the quality and vitality of the conversion. And it has always wanted to do everything to provide for an adequate formation of this faith—it has always wanted to, but this desire has often remained abstract, leaving a tragic contradiction between formal declarations and reality.

Structures

The preparation for baptism, at first very supple and rather rapid (first and second centuries), was soon realistically affirmed (second and third centuries). The second period, which seems to be representative, was characterized by the following:

— Evangelization, the proposal of the Christian message to men and women of good will, preceded the catechumenate.
— But good will is not enough: the entry into the catechumenate was open only to those who had made the step of conversion to Christ. Only a believer could have access to catechesis.
— Catechesis, the purpose of which was both doctrinal and vital, necessarily endured for a rather long time.
— During the course of this slow formation, the candidate was already a member of the Church in a certain way by virtue of the recognized conversion. Thus the Fathers called the candidate already a Christian.[74] Certain sacramentals could be received since God nourishes his children throughout this period of gestation.

— The catechumenate was a community in which the faith grew over several years. The catechumens had the time to find their place, to live in it, and to grow.

— The sacramental act, however, was not completed until after the examination of the aptitude of the candidate that inaugurated the period of solemn admission to baptism.

Historically, the authenticity of this pastoral perspective achieved its optimum form during the three centuries when the Church was doing missionary work in a hostile world. When the Church was recognized officially, it was forced to confront a new social context and hardly knew how to adapt. Everyone who was associated with it became the "Church." And, burdened with this Christian environment that gave the impression that the Church had arrived at the end of its journey, it lost the evangelical vigor of its faith.[75] It was no longer capable of bringing about conversion or of sustaining the journey of the catechumens to the eucharist.

Whether we are concerned with a young Church or a Church already matured by the centuries, it is always necessary to safeguard the traditional spirit of a serious and progressive catechumenal formation. The modes may change, and indeed they must be adapted to the concrete historical situation. But the journey of the individual to his or her Lord must be respected, just as the Lord has respected it to approach us.

Notes

[1] Cf H. Tardif, *Catéchuménat d'hier et d'aujourd'hui,* Masses ouvrières (12 avenue Sainte-Rosalie, Paris XIII) 142 , June 1958, pp. 45-62; *Etapes catéchuménales,* Masses ouvrières 137, January 1958, pp. 13-24. These works nuance the affirmations of very rapid baptism in the absence of the catechumenate.

[2] Cyril of Jerusalem, *Selections from the Catechetical Lectures,* ed. by William Telfer, *The Library of Christian Classics IV: Cyril of Jerusalem and Nemesius of Emesa. Procatechesis,* 17,35-36.

[3] Ambrose, *In Psalm.* 118, 20. 48-9, PL 15,1499, A to C.

[4] Ibid.

[5] Augustine, *Serm.* 47,17.

[6] Augustine, *De catechizandis rudibus,* V,9: *The First Catechetical Instruction,* trans. by Joseph P. Christopher, ACW, p. 24.

[7] Augustine, *Confessions,* 1,1,11.

[8] *Exp. in Luc.* 4,76: SC 45(2), ed. by G. Tissot, 1971, p.181.

[9] Basil, *Hom. XIII sur le Saint Baptême,* I,3,7, PG 31, 425 ff. (preached in 371).

[10] *Sermon sur le Saint Baptême,* orat. 40, nr. 11, PG 36, 372 B-C (preached in 381).

[11] PG 45, 416-32.

[12] *Quaest. ad Simpl.* 1,2,2, PL 40,111-2. Augustine takes the example of catechumens to illustrate his thesis: "Man begins to receive grace from the moment when he begins to believe in God, since he is moved toward the faith by an interior or exterior motion."

[13] PG 59,115. John Chrysostom, *Baptismal Instructions,* trans. by Paul W. Harkins, ACW, 31, p. 179.

[14] PG 60, 23-5.

[15] Cf. M.-D. Chenu, "Foi et sacrement," *La Maison-Dieu* 71, pp. 69-77; L. Villette, *Foi et sacrement,* Paris, 1959, 1964; A. Monjardet, *Autre Eglise, autre foi,* L'Epi, Paris, 1967, pp. 171-88; P. Gerbe and E. Marcus, *Ils demandent le baptême pour leur enfant.* Le Cerf, Paris, 1966; see also J. Frisque, A. Laurentin, E. Marcus, J. Massaut, T. Maertens, and E. Potel, *Foi et sacrement, la sacramentalisation des non-pratiquants,* Coll. de Pastorale liturgique, 62, Biblica, Bruges, 1964, which includes a bibliographical bulletin on the problem of faith and sacrament by A. Laurentin, pp. 53-68.

[16] De Spiritu Sancto, 12,28; SC 17, p. 157. *Basil the Great on the Holy Spirit,* trans. by George Lewis, London, Religious Tract Society, s.d.

[17] PG 29,655.

[18]Athanasius, *IIe Or. adv. Ar.* nr. 3, PG 26,237, A-B.

[19]PG 26, 218.

[20]*Quaest. ad Simpl.* 1,2,2, PL 40,111-2.

[21]*De fide et op.* 1,1; FC, 27, p. 221.

[22]Ibid., 26,48. On the magical notion of the efficacy of baptism, cf. these words of Augustine: "They believe they can permit themselves to commit adultery, under the pretext that they are catechumens and they dare to appeal to the adulterous woman of the Gospels 'who was not condemned.' Let no one say *the adulterous woman obtained pardon and I am still a catechumen, I shall commit adultery because I shall be pardoned,*" Serm. 20,6; ed. G. Morin, *Miscellanea Agostiniana,* p. 116; cf. also *Serm.* 16 A, CCL 41, p. 222.

[23]*Procatechesis,* 1-2,4. PG 33, 1050ff.; SC 126.

[24]*IIe Hom. ad Illum.,* PG 49,234 (Antioch, Lent 388). English text partially from *John Chrysostom: Baptismal Instructions,* trans. by Paul W. Harkins, ACW 31, p. 179.

[25]*Or. Cat.* 40, PG 45,101, B-D, cf. 104 A. *The Catechetical Oration of St. Gregory of Nyssa,* trans. by J. H. Srawley, London, SPCK, 1917, p. 117.

[26]*Serm.* 200,2; CCL 104,808. *Saint Caesarius of Arles: Sermons, Vol. III,* trans. by Sr. Mary Magdeleine Mueller, OSF, FC 66, p. 59.

[27]*De fide et op.,* 5,7.

[28]Pseudo-Origen, Treatise XII of the edition of P. Batiffol and A. Wilmart, *Tractatus Origenis de libris SS. Scripturarum,* Paris, 1900, p. 135. On the image of Noah's ark applied to the Church in function of the catechumenate as Tertullian uses it, cf. Dujarier, *Parrainage des adultes,* p. 224.

[29]Cited in Hamman, *La Messe* (Lettres chrétiennes), p. 233; see also p. 240: "You have been sifted by fasts, meditations, vigils, exorcisms. You have been ground by exorcising; one does not knead without water; you have been baptized."

[30]John Chrysostom, *In Ep. I ad Cor. in Hom.* 12,7; PG 61, 106; Mark the Deacon, *Life of Porphyry of Gaza,* 6,45, PG 65, 1242; cf. trans. of H. Grégoire and M.A. Kugener, Paris, 1930, *Etudes byzantines,* pp. 37-8 and 118 (end 4th century). Most of the Fathers of the Church that we know of from the 4th century were inscribed in the catechumenate as children and baptized as adults after having been personally converted, thus Basil, Gregory of Nazianzus, Augustine, John Crysostom.

[31]Augustine, *Conf.,* 1,1,11; PL 32,668. *De cat. rud.* 26,50.

[32]*Vie de Porphyre,* 4,29, PG 65, 1226; cf. the trans. of H. Grégoire and M. A. Kugener, Paris, 1930, pp. 26-27, Ambrose, *In Psalm.* 118, PL 20, 168. One finds many conversions of this kind in the life of St. Martin by Sulpicius Severus, SC 133, pp. 283, 285, 291; also *Dial.* 11,4,9, PL 20, 204.

[33]B. Botte, "Les plus anciennes collections canoniques," *L'Orient syrien* 5, 1960. 331-50. *Canon d'Hippolyte,* text and trans. by R.-J.

Coquin, PO 31, pp. 273-444.

[34]*De cat. rud.* 26,50.

[35]Augustine, *Contra Cresc.*, 2,5,7.

[36]*De cat. rud.* 8,12: "If a candidate comes to you who has already cultivated classical studies . . . it is highly improbable that he does not know many passages of our Scriptures."

[37]Ibid. 5,9.

[38]Canon 42, Hefele, *Histoire des conciles* I, pp. 212 ff.

[39]This is the case, for example, with Marius Victorinus of whom Augustine speaks in *Conf.* 8,2,5.

[40]*De fide et op.,* 6,9; FC 27, p. 23.

[41]Cyril of Jerusalem, *Procatechesis,* 4 & 6; *Library of Christian Classics* 4.

[42]*I[e] Cat. ad Illum.* 4, PG 49,221 (Antioch, Lent, 387). LC 5, pp.179-80.

[43]*IIe Cat. ad Illum.*PG 49, 221; c. 231 (Antioch, Lent, 387), LC 5, p. 185.

[44]*Journal,* 45; SC 21, ed. H. Pétré, 1948, pp. 255-7; *Egeria's Travels,* trans. by John Wilkinson, London, SPCK, 1971, pp. 143-4.

[45]Theodore of Mopsuestia, *Hom. XII* (1st on Baptism), nr. 14; in *Les Homélies catéchétiques de Théodore de Mopsueste,* ST 145, 1949.

[46]L. Roques, *Le Parrainage des adultes d'après les homélies de Théodore de Mopsueste,* Inst. Sup. Past. Cat., Paris, 1961; V.S. Janeras, "En quels jours furent prononcées les homélies catéchétiques de Théodore de Mopsueste?" in *Memorial Mgr. Gabriel Khouri-Sarkis,* Leuven, 1969, pp. 121-33.

[47]In *Serm.* 200,2 (CCL 104,808), St. Caesarius states that the inscription of the name is done "several days before Easter," that is, a short time in advance.

[48]Canon 19, PO 31, 377.

[49]*Journal,* 46; SC 21, pp. 257-9; *Egeria's Travels,* pp. 144-5.

[50]The principal points of catechesis on the Creed are cited in my series of articles, "Pour une mise en oeuvre du nouveau rituel de l'initiation chrétienne des adultes," "Document 3: Les traditions" (in *Le Calao* 39, p. L 39, note 3).

[51]For the catechesis on the Our Father, ibid., p. L 40, note 5.

[52]*Journal,* 46. On the custom of the transmission of the Symbol and of the Our Father and of the submission to the Symbol at Hippo, see S. Poque, "Augustine d'Hippone: Sermons pour la Pâque," SC 116, pp. 59-69. The dates vary according to the Churches; see my article cited in note 50 above, pp. L 29- L 32.

[53]*De Symb.* 3,1,3; CCL 60,349.

[54]*Serm.* 216,6-7. On the manner of performing the scrutinies, see my article "Document 4: Les scrutins," in *Le Calao* 40, pp. L 42-L 45.

[55]*Hom. XIII,* 13,17, & 19. R. Tonneau and R. Devreesse, *Les homélies catéchétiques de Théodore de Mopsueste",* ST 145, pp. 391-401.

[56]In 385, in his *Epistle to Himerius of Tarragona,* Pope Siricius (384-

399) states that an ancient Roman custom recommends that adults only be baptized at Easter and in the period of joy up till Pentecost except in danger of death; *Ep.* I, 3, PL 13, 1134-1135; cf. *Ap. Trad.*, nr. 22 ff. See also Tertullian, *De bapt.* 19,1-3; CCL 1,293, and St. Leo, pope, Letter 16, 1-5 addressed to the Bishops of Sicily, 21 Oct. 447, LC 5, pp. 282-7.

[57]On this subject, see Jean Daniélou, *Bible et liturgie,* 1958, pp. 29-96, and my series of articles in *Le Calao* cited above. All these articles will appear in my book to be published by W.H. Sadlier Inc.: *The Rites of Christian Initiation of Adults, Historical and Pastoral Reflections,* (1979).

[58]John Chrysostom, *Cat. ad Illum.* 2,27 (Antioch, shortly after 388), SC 50, pp. 148-9.

[59]*Ibid.,* 4, 1, SC 50, p. 182.

[60]On the distinction between catechumen and the faithful, see my article "Qu'est-ce qu'un catéchumène? Recherche sur le statut du catéchumène dans l'Eglise," in *Le Calao,* 25 (1974,1), pp. 22-5.

[61]John Chrysostom,*IIe Cat. ad Illum.,* 1; LC 5, p. 187. Also note the names "newly illuminated " (p. 187) and "neophyte" (p. 201) given to the newly baptized.

[62]Journal, 47; SC 21, p. 261; *Egeria's Travels,* pp. 145-6.

[63]Cf. my article, "Le temps du néophytat" to be published in *Le Calao* 47, particularly note 12.

[64]John Chrysostom, *Cat.* 4, 4; SC 50(2), p. 184.

[65]Ibid., 5,20; SC 50(2), p. 210.

[66]Ibid., 4 ,17; SC 50(2), pp. 191-3. See also 18-19.

[67]*Hom. in Act. Ap.,* 1,8; PG 60 cc. 24-25 (Constantinople, Lent, 400).

[68]*Sermon on Holy Baptism,* 13; PG 36, 373 D; 376 A; ES, p. 72; LC 5, p. 119.

[69]Cf. "Epistle to Diognetus," 5-6.

[70]The reduction of the catechumenate to the Lenten period marks the beginning of major decline. See Appendix II below.

[71]At the time of Caesarius, the parents had to bring their babies who were to be baptized at Easter to the Lenten catechumenal ceremonies. But already, some mothers tried to avoid this custom (*Serm.* 84,6). On the subject of the evolution of the baptismal rite under the influence of infant baptism, see P. Riche, "Education et culture dans l'occident barbare VIe-VIIIe siècles." *Patristica sorboniensa* 4, Paris, 1962, pp. 532-5, and J.-Ch. Didier, "Une adaptation de la liturgie baptismale au baptême des enfants dans l'Eglise ancienne." *Mélanges de sciences religieuses* 22, 1965, pp. 79-90.

[72]Cf. M. Dujarier, "Le Catéchuménat et la maternité de l'Eglise," *La Maison-Dieu* 71, pp. 78-93.

[73]This is why the Fathers so often used with regard to the catechumenate this saying of Christ: "Do not give dogs what is holy; and do not throw your pearls before swine" (Mt 7:6). See above Chap. 2, n. 4.

[74]Augustine, *Tract. in Jo.* 44, 2. Cf. also 11,3; *Serm.* 136,3, and the *Serm. ad catech.* published in *Revue bénédictine* 50, 1938, pp. 186-193 and also *Serm.* 294,14 in PLS 2, 192-5. See also my article cited in note 3, p. 57 above.

[75]On the use and the sense of the word "vigor" by the Christian writers of North Africa in the 3rd century, particularly St. Cyprian, see J. Daniélou, *Les origines du christianisme latin,* Cerf, Paris, 1978, pp. 349-55.

Appendix I:
Can a History
of the Catechumenate
Be Written?

General Survey

WHILE there are many studies on the baptismal liturgy, no exhaustive modern study tracing the history of the catechumenate has been published. Without attempting to give a complete bibliography on the subject, we compiled the following list of works that could aid in such a study.

The works of the sixteenth and nineteenth century are not to be set aside out of hand. Even if their documentation is less complete than that of modern studies, they often go into a great amount of detail.[1]

In the beginning of the twentieth century, the only study of any depth is the one contributed by Dom de Puniet to the *Dictionnaire d'Archéologie Chrétienne et de Liturgie*.[2] Even though it is dated, it is well-documented and can serve as a valuable reference. However, the discoveries of the last seventy years have rendered it largely obsolete. The reconstitution or publication of texts as valuable as *The Apostolic Tradition* of Hippolytus of Rome, the journal of Egeria, the homilies of Theodore of Mopsuestia and some of the catechetical sermons of St. John Chrysostom have thrown new light on the ancient catechumenate.

Much of the former work, however, dealt only with the liturgical aspects of baptism and gave little attention to the catechumenal practice itself. This is the case, for example, with the chapter L. Duchesne wrote on Christian initiation for his study on the origins of the Christian liturgy.[3]

More detailed studies of the history of the catechumenate did not appear in the following years. The survey that G. Bareille gives in the *Dictionnaire de Théologie Catholique*,[4] though very interesting, is not very extensive. And it is regrettable that recent dictionaries have given so little space to this traditional institution that could make a major contribution to modern pastoral renewal.[5]

Liturgical manuals, centered on the rites of baptism, do not delve very much into the history of the catechumenate.[6] When they do, they approach it through the great sacramentaries, that is, at a time when the liturgical rites no longer corresponded to actual practice.[7]

Nor do the major historical and juridical collections supply the information one has the right to expect from them. For the first three centuries, I note here only the article by Lebreton in Fliche and Martin's history of the Church[8] and Daniélou's treatment of the subject in his *Nouvelle Histoire de l'Eglise*.[9] For the fourth and fifth centuries, there is a chapter on the history of the law and the institutions of the Church in the West in Gaudemet's *L'Eglise dans l'Empire Romain*.[10]

I note with pleasure that over the last few years a number of works have appeared that complement the older studies on the baptismal ritual. First, there is the book by A. Stenzel, which devotes a large section to the rites of the catechumenate.[11] The book by T. Maertens is still too centered on the liturgical aspect alone and that too much from the Western point of view.[12] The very detailed study by C. Kretschmar is much richer and is also the best documented.[13]

Special Studies

WHILE waiting for a true history of the catechumenate, we can still profit from some good studies that deal with catechumenal practice in a specific period or region. The following list needs to be completed by systematic bibliographical research.

We shall first mention some editions of one or another work of ancient authors that, in the introductions, treat of baptismal preparation. In the collection *Sources Chrétiennes*, there are, for example:

B. Botte, "Hippolyte de Rome. La Tradition Apostolique," SC 11(2), pp. 28-9.

B. Botte, "Ambroise de Milan. Des Sacrements. Des Mystères. Explication du Symbole," SC 25(2), pp. 25-40.

F. Refoule, "Tertullien. Traité du Baptême," SC 35, pp. 29-45.

A. Wenger, "Jean Chrysostome. Huit Catéchèses Baptismales Inédites," SC 50(2), pp. 66-104.

S. Poque, "Augustin d'Hippone. Sermons pour la Pâque," SC 116, pp. 21-39.

J. Lemarie, "Chromace d'Aquilée. Sermons. Tome I," SC 154, pp. 87-103.

M.-J. Delage, "Césaire d'Arles. Sermons au Peuple. Tome I," SC 175, pp. 161-5.

M. Aubineau, "Hésychius de Jérusalem, Basile de Séleucie, Jean de Béryte, Pseudo-Chrysostome, Léonce de Constantinople. Homélies Pascales," SC 187.

There are numerous articles and works dealing with

a particular ancient author that bring out the catechumenal practice. For example:

For Tertullian:
E. Dekkers, *Tertullianus en de Geschiedenis der Liturgie*, Brugge, 1947, pp. 163-216.

For Ambrose:
B. Parodi, *La Catechesi di Sant'Ambrogio*, Gênes, 1957.
T.M. Peresson, "La Iniciacion Cristiana en el Testimonio de San Ambrosio de Milan," thesis, mimeograph in 2 volumes, Paris, s.d.
A. Caprioli, "Battesimo e Confermazione. Studio Storico sulla Liturgia e Catechesi di S. Ambrogio," Varese, 1977 (thesis for the Gregorian University).

For John Chrysostom:
T.M. Finn, *The Liturgy of Baptism in the Baptismal Instructions of St. John Chrysostom*, Washington, 1967.

For Augustine:
B. Busch, "De Initiatione Christiana secundum Doctrinam sancti Augustini," Vatican, 1939.
F. Van der Meer, *Saint Augustin Pasteur d'Âmes*, Colmar, 1955, vol. 2, pp. 113-69.
R. de Latte, *Saint Augustin et le Baptême. Etude Liturgico-Historique du Rituel Baptismal des Adultes chez Saint Augustin, Questions Liturgiques*, 1976, pp. 177-223.

Of particular interest are the studies that deal on a larger scale with an entire epoch or an entire region. Among others:

B. Capelle, "L'Introduction du Catéchuménat à Rome," *Recherches de Théologie Ancienne et Médiévale* 5, 1933, pp. 129-54.

126

A. Freitag, "Die Erziehung der Taufkandidaten im altchristlichen Katechumenat," *Zeitschrift für Missionswissenschaft* 17 (1927), pp. 174-94.

A. Bludau, "Das Katechumenat in Jerusalem im 4. Jahrhundert," *Theologie und Glaube* 16 (1924), pp. 225-42.

C. Garcia Del Valle, *Jerusalem, un Siglo de Oro de Vida Litúrgica*, Madrid 1968, pp. 65-140.

V. Monachino, *S. Ambrogio e la Cura Pastorale a Milano, Cartagine e Roma nel Secolo Quarto*, Rome, 1947.

P. Rentinck, *La Cura Pastorale in Antiochia nel 4° Sec.*, Rome, 1970, pp. 17-56.

V. Saxer, *Vie Liturgique et Quotidienne à Carthage vers le Milieu du 3ᵉ Siècle. Le Temoignage de S. Cyprien et de ses Contemporains d'Afrique*, Vatican, 1969, pp. 106-44.

J.-L. Duffes and C. Geay, *Le Baptême dans l'Eglise Copte*, Cairo, 1973, Book I, pp. 1-75.

H.M. Riley, *Christian Initiation. A Comparative Study of the Interpretation of the Baptismal Liturgy in the Mystagogical Writings of Cyril of Jerusalem, John Chrysostom, Theodore of Mopsuestia and Ambrose of Milan*, Washington, 1974.

T.C. Akeley, *Christian Initiation in Spain c. 300-1100*, London, 1967.

J.D.C. Fisher, *Christian Initiation, Baptism in the Medieval West: A Study in the Disintegration of the Primitive Rites of Initiation*, London, 1965.

L.L. Mitchell, *Baptismal Anointing*, London, 1966.

E.C. Whitaker, *Documents of the Baptismal Liturgy*, London, 2nd ed., 1970.

Many of the older studies on the catechumenate tended to devote too much time to the fourth and fifth centuries to the detriment of the preceding centuries.

It is true that this period is rich in catechetical documents and easily passes for a golden age of catechesis. But it would be wrong to make it a golden age of the catechumenate. Though "catechumens" were still numerous, the catechumenal framework had become lax and only existed during Lent.

It was during the third century that the journey toward baptism was the most demanding and the best structured, as is shown by what Hippolytus of Rome writes. But historians have yet to demonstrate that the Hippolytian practice was not a happy exception and does indeed reflect the customary way of doing things throughout the Mediterranean world. A more profound examination of this period is therefore necessary to construct the true picture of the catechumenal stages.[14]

Finally, research must be extended to include the first century. The pastoral practice of the very early Church, though it did not yet include the institution of the catechumenate in the strict sense, does reveal a concern for authenticity in baptismal preparation that forms the basis of the requirements of the later discipline.[15]

Notes

1. Among the many works available, I mention only the two following works in French:

   C. Chardon, *Histoire des sacraments, Paris, 1745, Vol. I, pp. 4-153,* "Des preparations au baptême, ou du catéchuménat."

   J. Corblet, *Histoire dogmatique, liturgique et archéologique du sacrement de baptême,* Paris, Vol. I (1881), pp. 443-74: "De la préparation au baptême." In his second volume (1882), pp. 583-92, he gives a very extensive bibliography of works in all languages relative to baptism that were published from the 16th to the 19th century.

2. P. de Puniet, "Catéchuménat," *Dictionnaire d'archéologie chrétienne et de liturgie* II,2,Paris (1910), cols. 2579-2621. Cf. the bibliography that cites many works in German from the end of the 19th century, and particularly J. Mayer, *Geschichte des Katechumenats und der Katechese in den ersten sechs Jahrhunderten,* Kempten, 1868.

3. L. Duchesne, *Origines du culte chrétien,* 5th ed., 1920, pp. 309-60.

4. G. Bareille, "Catéchuménat," *Dictionnaire de théologie catholique,* Paris, II,2, cols. 1968-87.

5. For example, G. Bardy, "Catéchuménat," *Catholicisme,* Vol. 2, cols. 664-7.

6. The most interesting is that of M. Righetti , *Storia liturgica,* Milan, Vol. IV (1959), pp. 21-146: "Il Battesimo." We note, too, Beraudy, "L'Initiation chrétienne" in *L'Eglise en prière,* Paris, 3rd ed., 1965, pp. 534-43.

   Also worthy of interest but too limited in scope are the chapters written in the following four works:

   Communion solennelle et profession de foi, Paris, 1952, chap. I: "L'Initiation à Rome dans l'antiquité et le haut moyen-âge," pp. 14-32.

   J. Daniélou, *Bible et liturgie,* Paris, 2nd ed., 1958, chap. I: "La Préparation (au baptême)," pp. 29-49.

   J. Jungmann, *La Liturgie des premiers siècles,* Paris, 1962 chap. VII: "Le Baptême et la préparation au baptême," pp. 119-36 (see also pp. 382-6).

   A Benoit, "Le Baptême, sa célébration et sa signification dans L'Eglise ancienne," in *Baptême, Sacrement d'Unité,* Maine, 1971, pp. 9-84

7. In this regard, we cite:

   A. Crogaert, *Baptême, Confirmation, Eucharistie: Sacraments de L'initiation chrétienne,* Bruges-Paris, 1946.

H.A.P. Schmidt, *Introductio in liturgiam occidentalem,* Herder, 1960, chap. XIV: "Initiatio christiana," pp. 238-96.

A. Nocent, "Iniziazione cristiana," pro manuscripto, Rome, 1972, esp. pp. 203-335.

8. A. Fliche and V. Martin, *Histoire de l'Eglise,* Paris, Vol. I, 1938, pp. 263-5 and 366-7; Vol. II, 1943, pp. 66-9.

9. J. Daniélou and H. Marrou, *Nouvelle histoire de l'Eglise,* Vol. I, pp. 99-104 and 191-4.

10. J. Gaudemet, *L'Eglise dans l'empire romain (4°-5°s.),* Paris, 1958, pp. 56-68.

11. A. Stenzel, *Die Taufe,* Innsbruck, 1958.

12. T. Maertens, *Histoire et pastorale du rituel du catéchuménat et du baptême,* Bruges, 1962.

13. G. Kretschmar, "Die Geschichte des Taufgottesdienstes in der alten Kirchen," in *Leiturgia,* ed. 31-4, Kassel, 1964-1966.

14. M. Dujarier, *La Parrainage des adultes aux trois premiers siècles de l'Eglise,* Paris, 1962, pp. 177-344.

15. Ibid., pp. 71-171.

Appendix II:
Decline and Revival
of the Catechumenate:
Sixth to the
Twentieth Century

To better understand how the catechumenate of the first centuries of the Church can serve as a source for the current renewal of Christian initiation, let us examine the evolution of catechumenal practice from the sixth century to the present.[1]

The Eclipse of the Catechumenate

1. FIRST, we must stress that there was a kind of "catechumenate" for infants. It is interesting to note that, even for babies, the celebration of baptism was not limited to one single liturgical ceremony. The practice of the seven scrutinies on the weekdays of Lent developed when there were many infants among the candidates.[2] The testimony of Caesar of Arles in the sixth century is irrefutable: addressing himself to mothers bringing their babies to the scrutinies, he urged them not to miss these celebrations.[3] This custom was undoubtedly a vestige of the tradition of baptizing infants at the same time as adults. It shows that the normative rite of Christian initiation was baptism by stages, since the sacrament supposes faith and therefore progress in the faith.

   This custom also had the great advantage of having the parents of these infants participate in the preparation for baptism. Since the parents "answered" for their children, it was normal that they make the catechetical and liturgical journey leading to baptism.[4]

2. With the phenomenon of the increasing number and rapidity of adult baptisms in the mission areas, there were always voices raised demanding at least a minimum of serious preparation. Unfortunately, these appeals had little effect.[5]

   Following Pope Siricius (385) and Pope Leo the Great (447), the Council of Agde (506) and Pope

Gregory II (at the beginning of the eighth century) insisted that baptisms be celebrated only on the feasts of Easter and Pentecost. By thus reducing the number of celebrations, it was hoped that serious preparation could be more easily provided. Unfortunately, there were those who pleaded that it was urgent to convert the pagans and that there were far too few priests to limit the celebration of baptism to just two days a year.

In any case, what was most important was the provision of at least a minimal period of preparation. Among those who struggled for this reform were:

— Martin of Braga, the Apostle of Sueves, succeeded in having the Council of Braga (572) adopt a law requiring three weeks of preparation so that the catechumens would have the time to be instructed in the Creed.[6]

— Boniface, the famous apostle of Germany at the beginning of the eighth century, instructed his catechumens for at least two months, and even longer.[7]

— Alcuin, faced with the mass baptisms Charlemagne was imposing by force, succeeded in launching a certain catechumenal reform. Drawing upon Augustine's *De Catechizandis Rudibus*, Alcuin pressed for serious catechesis. In practical terms, he demanded a preparation of between seven days and forty days.[8]

Timid reforms, certainly, but in their context, they did signify real progress. Unfortunately, these attempts were quickly forgotten; even though they sometimes carried the weight of written Church law, they had little effect in the following centuries. But the attempt to reestablish catechumenal practice centuries later drew its inspiration from Martin of Braga before turning directly to the customs of the early Church.

3. During the Middle Ages, for all practical purposes the catechumenate no longer existed. Still there were some traces, very minimal ones, it is true, but ones that show that the catechumenal reality had not completely disappeared from the Church. Some of these traces can be found in theological thought and others in the liturgy.

In the twelfth century, Hugo of Saint Victor could still treat of the catechumenate in his "De Sacramentis Fidei Christiana."[9] In the following century, St. Thomas mentioned "catechumens" several times in his *Questiones* on baptism.[10] Unfortunately, in the mission areas, mass baptisms were administered after only a few days of preparation.

Elements of the ancient catechumenal stages were also preserved in the rituals of this period. But more and more they were mixed together and celebrated in one single ceremony. They did exist, but as witnesses that had lost their significance at the same time as their application.

Modern Missionary Efforts

BETWEEN the sixteenth and the twentieth centuries, an authentic movement to recover the catechumenate developed.[11] Everywhere that the Gospel was preached by the missionaries, a very strong spirit of reform attempted to restore catechumenal preparation. There was much enthusiasm, but it encountered strong resistance. To succeed, almost five centuries of constant effort were necessary. These efforts, like successive waves, washed over Latin America, then Asia, and then Africa before finally returning to old Europe. Let us briefly consider how three successive reforms culminated in the renewal of the catechumenate.

Sixteenth Century

Latin America. From the 1500's onwards, the Franciscans, under pressure from the civil authorities, directed their attention primarily to mass conversion. Indians were baptized by the tens of thousands without much preparation. The Dominican and Augustinian missionaries began to counteract this situation upon their arrival in Latin America in 1526. In 1534, the Augustinians requested that baptisms be celebrated only four times a year: at Easter, Pentecost, the Feast of St. Augustine, and the Epiphany. In 1538, an episcopal conference urged pastors to return to the missionary principles of Alcuin and required a catechumenate of forty days that included fasting, catechesis, exorcisms, and scrutinies. But these proposals never found their way into general practice and provincial synods found it necessary to repeat them in 1585.

Asia and Africa. The same tendency of quick and easy baptism existed in Central Africa and in the first missions of Asia. St. Francis Xavier, at the beginning of his apostolate, baptized great numbers of people very quickly. But it was impossible to ignore the fact that many of the neophytes just as rapidly abandoned the Christian faith.

In reaction, St. Ignatius Loyola, in 1552, successfully urged the establishment in India of catechumenal houses where the converts gathered for three months of baptismal preparation. It was also at this time that the first catechisms appeared. There were those, to be sure, who opposed Ignatius in this matter, but the bishops succeeded in establishing this discipline.

The Seventeenth and Eighteenth Centuries

Though the victory had yet to be won, the battle had been joined. Many liturgists and missionaries tried to solidify the base of the renewal and to extend its practice.

Some Notable Proponents of the Renewal.[12] Cardinal Julius Anthony Sanctorius, a close aide of Pius V and later of Gregory XIII and Clement VIII, did extensive research on ancient liturgies. After twenty-five years of study, he published in 1602 a book entitled *Restored Roman Ritual Based on the Practice of the Ancient Church.* In it, the baptismal liturgy was extended throughout the duration of the catechumenate. This ritual of 712 pages was never promulgated, though it was distributed to the members of the commission responsible for drawing up a ritual.

It was a Carmelite by the name of Thomas of Jesus who, sensitive to the needs of the apostolate, brought Sanctorius's work to wider attention. In 1613 he published a weighty tome of 926 pages entitled *On the Manner of Procuring Salvation for All Pagans* that took up the project of Sanctorius and added practical suggestions for the catechesis of catechumens and even neophytes.

The efforts to establish a catechumenal pedagogy in Asia were particularly significant, but they lacked a liturgical dimension. The Congregation for the Propagation of the Faith, founded in 1622, distributed the work of Thomas of Jesus to the missionaries leaving for Asia. At that time, the *Missions Etrangères* of Paris began to issue their "Instructions," which gave very practical advice for the realization of an authentic catechumenal initiation.

These developments formed the basis for the young Asian Churches to establish a progressive journey through the stages of initiating the catechumens into the faith. Unfortunately, the liturgical renewal did not include any stages. True, certain signs were used to mark ceremonially the passage along the journey to baptism, but they were not liturgical rites properly speaking. And finally, this progressive pedagogy gradually faded away in the nineteenth century, faithful though it was to the tradition of the Church and to the needs of the pastoral situation.

The Nineteenth and Twentieth Centuries

In Africa the century-old effort for the renewal of the catechumenate was relaunched. It was a renewal whose results have now been realized throughout the Universal Church, thanks to the perseverance of generations of missionaries in the four corners of the world.

From the eighteenth century on, the Capuchins and the Holy Ghost missionaries strove to restore baptismal preparation. But Cardinal Lavigerie deserves the credit for re-establishing a vigorous and traditional catechumenal discipline.[13] His pedagogy rested on two key elements: (1) preparation for baptism must be carried out in stages, each step marking a progression in catechesis and in conversion; (2) the preparation for baptism presupposes a certain length of time in order to assure an initiation that will lead to perseverance in the Christian life.

Practically speaking, these two principles led to the establishment of a period of postulancy (two years), followed by a period of the catechumenate (two years), and finally to a major baptismal retreat.

Unfortunately, these developments still lacked a proper liturgical dimension. The giving of medals, rosaries, or crucifixes was an attempt to signify the progress of the catechumens, but there were no liturgical stages signifying the progressive gift of divine grace. Restoration of the liturgical dimension would be the contribution of the old European continent, only lately awakened to catechumenal pedagogy.

It was the example of the African catechumenate that roused the Churches of Europe.[14] Its most unique characteristic is the restoration, *ad experimentum*, of liturgical steps accompanying the journey of the catechumen.

The Conciliar Renewal

THE Church today is at a crucial turning point. The restoration of the catechumenate is something already accomplished and something yet to be done. Fundamental decisions have been taken and the plans have been made, but the real work remains.

Fundamental Decisions Were Taken on Two Occasions

First, the Sacred Congregation of Rites, without waiting for the immanent opening of the Second Vatican Council, published on 16 April 1962 a decree restoring the rite of baptism in stages. The ritual was divided into distinct stages that, in keeping with the ancient tradition of the Church, would sustain the catechumen throughout the course of his formation and his journey toward baptism. This revised ritual was authorized for use where the bishops deemed it necessary.

But the text was still that of the old ritual for the baptism of adults. The revised ordo simply divided the rite into seven parts, but did nothing to modify the rites and prayers, many of which were repetitive and not in their authentic order. Therefore, the decree of 1962, though significant insofar as it opened the door to renewal, made the need for reform of the ritual all the more obvious.

The Second Vatican Council affirmed and specified this fundamental decision. The Constitution on the Sacred Liturgy promulgated the restoration of the "catechumenate of adults comprising several distinct steps" (§64). The Decree on the Church's Missionary Activity presented the nature and the meaning of the different moments of the journey of Christian initiation (§§13 and 14). Other texts added further specifications:

- on the responsibility of the bishops to restore the catechumenate (Decree on the Bishops' Pastoral Office in the Church, §14);
- on the maternal role of the Church in catechumenal action (Dogmatic Constitution on the Church, §14);
- on the role of the community in the initiation of catechumens (Decree on the Ministry and Life of Priests, §6);
- on the reform of the ritual of Christian initiation (Constitution on the Sacred Liturgy, §§65 and 66).

The outlines of the work to be undertaken were proposed by the Commissions after consultation with the Churches. In 1966, the Commission on the Liturgy drew up a provisional ritual and distributed it for experimentation to the different Churches throughout the world. After an examination of the responses, the second draft was formulated and distributed in 1969 to elicit still more remarks and suggestions. The responses to this second draft formed the basis for the new *Rite of Christian Initiation of Adults,* which was promulgated on 6 January 1972.

Let's Get to Work!

The appearance of this new ritual does not put an end to the research into, and the development of, the catechumenate. Quite the contrary, it is an invitation to adaptation and creativity.[15]

It is a guide, not a recipe. Before using the new rite, it is necessary to plumb its spirit and to understand the theology it affirms and the pedagogical orientations it proposes. This is to say that it is a guide that permits different ways of application that are to be determined both by the culture of the people and by the concrete circumstances of their lives.

It is not a ritual to be translated but an instrument for creating a ritual. When it comes to liturgy and ritual, a valid "translation" demands adaptation, and true adaptation is, in reality, a new creation, for liturgy must spring from the hearts and the lives of those who celebrate it. This is why the introduction of the Ritual leaves a great deal to the initiative of the regional episcopal conferences, as well for the style of the prayers as for the choice of the most expressive rites.

Notes

1. This section is largely taken from my article published in *Becoming a Catholic Christian*, Sadlier, New York, 1978, pp. 14-18. Some additions have been made.
2. A. Chavasse, "Histoire de l'initiation chrétienne des enfants, de l'antiquité à nos jours," in *La Maison-Dieu*, nr. 28, p. 32.
3. Louise Bonnet, "Les Fonctions de parrainage d'après les homélies de St. Césaire d'Arles," memoire at the ISPC, Paris, 1968, pp. 33-40.
4. Especially Sermons 84, 225,6 and 229,6.
5. For this period and the following, cf:
   L. Kilger, "Zur Entwicklung der Katechumenatspraxis vom 5. bis 18. Jahrhundert," in *Zeitschrift für Missionswissenschaft* 15 (1925), pp. 166-82.
   G. Mensaert, "La Préparation des adultes au baptême en terre paienne," in *Revue d'histoire des missions* 16 (1939), especially pp. 250-5 and 510-4.
6. Migne Latin 84, 571.
7. F. Flaskamp, "Die Missionsmethode des hl. Bonifatius," in *Zeitschrift für Missionswissenschaft* 15 (1925), pp. 18-49, especially pp. 85-6.
8. Danube Synod in 796. On the catechetical effort of this period, see A. Etchegaray Cruz, "Le rôle du De catechizandis rudibus de Saint Augustin dans la catéchèse missionnaire dès 710 jusqu'a 847," in *Studia patristica* XI (T.U. 108), pp. 316-21.
9. Liber II, pars IV, cap. 9 (de catechizatione), Migne Latin 176, 455ff.
10. Especially IIIa, q 68, art 2, 3 et 4; et q 71, art I.
11. J. Beckmann, "L'Initiation et la célébration baptismale dans les missions, du XVI siècle à nos jours," in *La Maison-Dieu* nr. 58, pp. 48-70.
12. J. Christiaens, "L'organisation d'un catéchuménat au XVI siècle," in *La Maison-Dieu*, nr. 58, pp. 71-82.
13. J. Perraudin, "Le Catéchuménat d'après le Cardinal Lavigerie," in *Parole et mission*, nr. 14, pp. 386-95.
14. On the history of the renewal in France, see "Vers un catéchuménat d'adultes" in *Documentation catéchistique* 37 (July 1957) which was revised and expanded in "Problèmes du catéchuménat," supplement of *Catéchèse*, Paris, 1961. See also J. Vernette and H. Bourgeois, *Seront-ils chrétiens?* Paris, Châlet, 1975.
15. For example, see M. Dujarier, "Expériences d'initiation chrétienne en Afrique de l'Ouest," in *Concilium*, nr. 142 (1979), pp. 77-84.